María del Pilar Díaz Martínez

Basic principles of the physiotherapist in dry needling

María del Pilar Díaz Martínez

Basic principles of the physiotherapist in dry needling

Key fundamentals for the effective application of dry needling

ScienciaScripts

Imprint
Any brand names and product names mentioned in this book are subject to trademark, brand or patent protection and are trademarks or registered trademarks of their respective holders. The use of brand names, product names, common names, trade names, product descriptions etc. even without a particular marking in this work is in no way to be construed to mean that such names may be regarded as unrestricted in respect of trademark and brand protection legislation and could thus be used by anyone.

Cover image: www.ingimage.com

This book is a translation from the original published under ISBN 978-613-9-44232-4.

Publisher:
Sciencia Scripts
is a trademark of
Dodo Books Indian Ocean Ltd. and OmniScriptum S.R.L publishing group

120 High Road, East Finchley, London, N2 9ED, United Kingdom
Str. Armeneasca 28/1, office 1, Chisinau MD-2012, Republic of Moldova, Europe
Managing Directors: Ieva Konstantinova, Victoria Ursu
info@omniscriptum.com

Printed at: see last page
ISBN: 978-620-8-60904-7

Copyright © María del Pilar Díaz Martínez
Copyright © 2025 Dodo Books Indian Ocean Ltd. and OmniScriptum S.R.L publishing group

CONTENTS

1. INTRODUCTION TO TRIGGER POINTS (PG)

1.1. History and definition of trigger points (TP).

The understanding of musculoskeletal pain has advanced significantly, focusing on identifying specific sources and causes, such as neuropathic, joint dysfunction, muscular causes and pain modulation by the central nervous system. The history of muscle pain was extensively reviewed during the 20th century and recently updated, highlighting the publications that underpin our current understanding of trigger point (TP) myofascial pain.

In the 19th century, Froriep described "Muskel Sch wiele" as palpable and painful hardnesses in the muscles, while Adler in America used the term "muscular rheumatism" and introduced the concept of pain radiating from tender points. In England, Gowers, Stockman and Llewellyn Jones introduced the term "fibrositis", while in Germany, Schmidt used "Muskelrheumatismus". Schade, in 1919, found that muscle stiffness persisted even after death, suggesting that the cause was not active muscle contraction, and proposed the term "Myogelosen". During the following decades, several researchers, such as F. Lange and M. Lange, contributed to the understanding of muscle responses and PGs. In 1937, Hans Kraus first used ethyl chloride spray to treat "Muskelhiirten" and subsequently PGs. Kellgren, in 1938, demonstrated referred pain patterns by injecting saline into muscles. In this same period, three physicians, Michael Gutstein, Michael Kelly and Janet Travell, identified myofascial PGs in different regions of the world, each using different diagnostic terms, but describing similar characteristics such as palpable hardness, points of extreme tenderness, referred pain and relief by massage or infiltration. Travell, in particular, had a lasting influence with over 40 articles published between 1942 and 1990, and his "Manual of Trigger Points" published in 1983 and 1992, where he documented PG pain patterns in 32 skeletal muscles (1).

Pathologic studies have attempted to identify the cause of PGs. Miehlke and colleagues conducted an extensive study on fibrositis, finding dystrophic findings in more symptomatic cases. The relationship between fibromyalgia and PGs has been a matter of debate, but in 1990, a group of rheumatologists established diagnostic criteria for fibromyalgia, linking it to central nervous system dysfunction. In the mid-1980s, A. Fischer developed a pressure algometer to measure PG sensitivity and hypersensitive points in fibromyalgia (1).

Finally, recent needle EMG studies by Hubbard and Berkoff in 1993 and rabbit experiments by Hong and Torigoe in 1994 confirmed that a dysfunctional motor plate area is the main location of PG pathophysiology. An additional advance was the interexaminer reliability study by Gerwin in 1994, which demonstrated reliable identification of myofascial PG criteria in five muscles (1).

With respect to the definitions that can be found, myofascial pain syndrome (MPS) is a condition characterized by a set of sensory, motor and autonomic signs and symptoms resulting from the presence of myofascial trigger points (MTrPs). These MTrPs are hyperirritable areas within a tight band of skeletal muscle, which present as palpable nodules and are painful when pressed, stretched or contracted (6). In addition to localized pain, PGMs can cause referred pain, motor dysfunction, and autonomic phenomena, such as changes in skin temperature or abnormal sweating and have a diameter between 2 and 5 mm. To diagnose MDS, it is crucial to identify all PGMs that contribute to symptoms, even if some of them are not clinically active. MDS can affect a single muscle (monomuscular MDS) or involve larger muscle groups or anatomical regions (2).

The concept of MTrPs has evolved since the term was introduced by orthopedic surgeon A. Steindler in 1940, who observed that novocaine infiltrations of these points relieved certain muscle pain. However, the most commonly used definition for trigger points is provided by Janet Travell and David Simons in 1992 "A myofascial trigger point (MTrP) is a muscle point that is extremely irritable, associated with a palpable hypersensitive nodule within a tight band". They were among the pioneers in researching and publishing on MTrPs, developing a manual that has become a reference for subsequent studies. Historically, PGMs have been known by various names, which has led to confusion. However, the terminology developed by Travell and Simons has been widely accepted in the scientific community. These trigger points, when found in skeletal muscles, can trigger referred pain, hypersensitivity and dysfunction, making accurate diagnosis and appropriate treatment essential (3).

1.2. Importance and epidemiology of PGs.

The skeletal musculature, the largest organ of the human body and accounting for almost 50% of body weight, is made up of approximately 400 muscles. These muscles can develop myofascial trigger points (TTPs) that cause pain and motor dysfunction, sometimes radiating to other areas. It cannot be stated that all painful points to the touch are MTPs, to consider it a trigger point we must observe other characteristics that will be detailed later in the section on trigger point diagnosis. This type of pain complicates diagnosis and can lead to inadequate treatment. At least 30% of the population experiences muscular symptoms, and many cases correspond to myofascial syndrome (MFS), a common but underdiagnosed problem, especially because it does not always present visible alterations in imaging tests or analysis (4).

MFS is a disabling condition, especially in the working age population, and although it is treatable, its effective management requires not only pain relief, but also correction of structural and postural problems. The correct diagnosis and treatment of this condition is crucial to improve the quality of life of patients (5). MPS is related to various musculoskeletal complaints such as low back pain (6), cervical pain (7), headaches (8, 9) or scapular pain (10). MMPs can be either the primary cause of pain or a secondary complication of other pathologies. Although myofascial pain is not life-threatening, it can severely affect quality of life.

It is essential to differentiate MFS from other disorders, such as fibromyalgia, because although they share certain symptoms, their treatments are different. Fibromyalgia, which is a different condition from MDS, has been linked to MDS because of the similarity in some of its symptoms. Fibromyalgia is characterized by a central sensitization process that causes widespread pain in various tissues, including muscles. In order to advance fibromyalgia research and to facilitate its diagnosis and classification, 18 specific pressure pain points have been identified, most of which overlap with myofascial trigger points. This overlap, together with the lack of knowledge of MDS and the difficulties in diagnosing it, has led to confusion and misdiagnosis. It is very common for people with fibromyalgia to also have MDS, but it does not occur with the same frequency in the reverse direction (11).

The cost associated with myofascial pain is high and mostly avoidable. Many people suffer persistent pain that could improve with proper diagnosis and treatment. Failure to recognize the myofascial nature of pain leads to misdiagnosis, creating frustration and hindering effective treatment. It is crucial that healthcare professionals improve their training and understanding of myofascial PGs to reduce the suffering and costs associated with untreated chronic pain. In addition, increasing research and outreach about this condition can optimize treatments and improve patients' quality of life (11).

With respect to epidemiology, myofascial trigger points (TP) are extremely common and affect a large percentage of the population. In a study of 200 asymptomatic young adults, 54% of women and 45% of men were found to have PGs in the muscles of the shoulder girdle. In addition, 25% of these subjects with latent PGs experienced pain referred. In another study of 269 nursing students, PGs were identified in 54% of the right lateral pterygoid muscles, 45% of the right deep right masseter muscles, 43% of the anterior part of the right temporalis, and 40% of the right medial pterygoid muscles. As for the neck muscles, 35% of the head splenius and 33% of the right trapezius showed PG. A neurologist examined 96 patients in a pain clinic and found that in 93% of cases, at least part of the pain was caused by myofascial PGs, being the primary cause of pain in 74% of these patients. Furthermore, in an orthopedic clinic, 21% of patients with musculoskeletal pain had active PGs in the pyramidal muscle (12).

Data show that myofascial PGs are a significant source of pain and dysfunction, with prevalence varying among different studies and populations. However, these trigger points remain underdiagnosed due to a lack of clear diagnostic criteria and insufficient training in this field. This contributes to incorrect diagnoses and unnecessary suffering for patients, in addition to high economic costs due to lost productivity and inadequate treatments. In summary, myofascial PGs affect a significant percentage of the population and are one of the leading causes of musculoskeletal pain, underscoring the need for a greater focus on their diagnosis and proper treatment in clinical practice (12).

1.3. Characteristics, types and formation mechanism of PGs.

The following are the key clinical features of myofascial trigger points (MTrPs) that physical therapists should recognize for the diagnosis of myofascial trigger point syndrome (MTS) (13):

- Tension and tight band: Muscles with a PGM feel tight to palpation, especially compared to the healthy opposite side. This tightness is due to the presence of tight bands in the affected muscle. The taut band is a distinctive feature of PGM, although it can be difficult to identify in deep muscles or muscles with excess fat.
- Focality of pain: On palpation of the taut band, a specific point is identified that is noticeably painful, known as the PGM. Moderate pressure on this point can elicit an intense painful response, known as the jump sign. This sign indicates high sensitivity at the PGM, although its variability and subjectivity make it less reliable in studies, with algometry being a more accurate tool for measuring pain threshold.
- Local twitch response: The local twitch response (REL) is observed when the PGM is pinched or when rapid palpation is performed. It consists of a rapid contraction of the fibers in the tense band, while the rest of the muscle remains relaxed. Although it is an important feature, it is not considered an essential diagnostic criterion due to its difficulty to obtain and variable reliability.
- Referred pain: Prolonged pressure on a PGM can cause referred pain to other areas of the body, following patterns specific to each PGM. Although these patterns are consistent, they are not universal and may vary. The ability to cause referred pain is variable and is not always a reliable diagnostic criterion, with puncture of the TMP being more effective in inducing referred pain compared to palpation.

- Stiffness and shortening: PGMs cause stiffness at rest and shortening of the affected muscle, which can limit joint mobility and cause pain when the muscle is stretched.
- Weakness and pain on contraction: Muscles with PGMs may experience weakness without atrophy, probably due to central inhibition. Electromyography shows that these muscles fatigue more easily and have a slower recovery after exercise. Muscle contraction tends to be more painful when the muscle is shortened.
- Activating mechanism: PGMs can be activated by direct mechanisms (such as trauma or overload) or indirect mechanisms (such as other PGMs, visceral diseases, or stress). Identifying these mechanisms can help in the diagnosis of MDS.

These clinical features are fundamental to the diagnosis and treatment of myofascial trigger points and may vary in presentation between individuals.

Muscle trigger points are hypersensitive areas within a skeletal muscle that, when pressed, cause local pain and often referred pain in other areas of the body. They are classified in various ways according to their activity, origin and clinical behavior. The main types of muscle trigger points are detailed below (14, 15).

1.3.1. According to its activity.

- Active trigger points: They are the direct cause of pain. They are those that cause spontaneous and constant pain, even without pressure or stimulus. These trigger points are the direct cause of the pain and are usually associated with a decrease in the functionality of the affected muscle. When pressed, they reproduce the referred pain and can trigger a muscle spasm response. Active trigger points are responsible for myofascial pain syndrome and can cause significant muscle dysfunction (14, 15).
- Latent trigger points: These do not cause pain unless stimulated by pressure or specific muscle activity. Although they are not painful to the touch in a normal state, they can limit mobility and generate muscle

weakness. Latent trigger points can be activated in situations of stress, muscle overuse, injury or fatigue, becoming active trigger points. They are the most common and can remain latent for long periods of time (14, 15).

1.3.2. According to their origin:

- Primary trigger points: They develop independently and have no clear underlying cause. They are directly related to muscle overexertion, overuse, improper posture or trauma. These points are what initially trigger muscle pain and, if left untreated, can contribute to the development of other trigger points in neighboring muscles (14, 15).
- Secondary trigger points: They originate as a result of another condition or dysfunction, such as nerve entrapment, radiculopathy (nerve root irritation) or joint dysfunction. These points usually develop in response to muscle tension generated by the primary condition, and their treatment must include the underlying cause for complete recovery (14, 15).

1.3.3. According to their relationship with other trigger points.

- Satellite trigger points: These develop in areas near a primary trigger point that has been active for a long time without adequate treatment. As the primary trigger point remains active, it can generate excessive tension in nearby muscles, leading to the appearance of these satellite trigger points. It is important to treat both primary and satellite trigger points to achieve complete pain relief (14, 15).
- Associated trigger points: These trigger points are found in muscles that are functionally or biomechanically related to the muscle containing the primary trigger point. Associated trigger points may develop in response to compensatory overload of neighboring muscles in an attempt to relieve pain or dysfunction of the primary affected muscle (14, 15).

1.3.4. According to the type of pain generated.

- Central PGMs: They are located in the motor plate area of the muscle, where dysfunctional motor plates provoke an energy crisis. This dysfunction generates contraction nodes, which form a nodule within a taut band. These central trigger points are associated with sensitization of local nociceptors in the area, generating pain. It is important to note that these points appear in the region of the muscle where the motor plates, or motor points, are located (14, 15).

- Insertional PGMs: They appear in the areas of muscle insertion, where muscle fibers are anchored to tendons, aponeurosis or bones. The increased tension maintained in these fibers can cause enthesopathy, with inflammation and increased tenderness in the insertion area. This may be more evident in muscles that have sufficient separation between the myotendinous and tenoperiosteal junctions, resulting in the presence of two clearly differentiated insertional PGs (14, 15).

Myofascial pain can be caused by a variety of factors that may act in isolation or in combination. Understanding these factors is essential to properly address pain and prevent its persistence. The following are the main mechanisms of formation and their triggers:

1.3.5. Triggering factors.

- Acute Trauma: After significant trauma, such as an accident or injury, myofascial pain may occur if pain persists beyond the acute phase of recovery. Under normal circumstances, the pain should subside as the tissue heals. However, when it persists, it is important to consider the possibility of myofascial pain, characterized by trigger points in the affected muscles (16).
- Postural Abnormalities: Postures maintained during daily activities, such as reading, writing or performing work tasks, can induce muscle stress. Poor posture during these activities can cause tension in the muscles and activate trigger points. The accumulation of tension in certain postural positions can lead to the formation of tight bands in the muscles, which in turn can trigger myofascial pain (16).
- Mechanical Factors: Skeletal alterations, such as spinal deviations or joint problems, can cause changes in the muscles that attempt to compensate for these abnormalities. For example, misalignment of the spine can result in additional tension in the neck and back muscles, which can activate trigger points and cause pain (16).

- Traffic Accidents: People involved in motor vehicle accidents often suffer from myofascial pain due to the traumatic injuries and strain they experience during impact (17).

1.3.6. Common areas of affectation.

- Head, Neck, Shoulders, Hips and Lumbar Region: These areas are frequently affected by myofascial pain because the muscles in these regions are constantly working against gravity or performing repetitive movements. Muscles that maintain posture or participate in repetitive daily activities are at risk for developing trigger points (17).

1.3.7. Psychological factors.

- Stress and Depression: Prolonged stress and depression can affect muscles by causing prolonged tension. These conditions can trigger trigger points and myofascial pain by altering the way the body handles stress and tension (15).
- Sleep Disturbances: Lack of restful sleep can prevent adequate relaxation of the muscles, causing them to remain in a state of continuous tension. This can lead to the formation of trigger points and myofascial pain, as well as muscle hyperirritability (15).

1.3.8. Nutritional and endocrine factors.

- Nutritional Deficiencies: Deficiencies in essential vitamins, such as B1, B12, C and folic acid, and minerals such as calcium, potassium, iron and magnesium can contribute to the development of trigger points. Lack of these essential nutrients can affect muscle health and predispose to trigger point formation (15).
- Endocrine Disorders: Problems in thyroid metabolism or other endocrine dysfunctions can affect muscle function and contribute to myofascial pain. Hormonal disturbances can influence the way muscles respond to stress and strain, exacerbating myofascial pain (15).

1.3.9. Degenerative

With age, due to aging muscle tissues may lose elasticity and flexibility, making muscles more prone to develop PGMs. Age-related structural degeneration may also contribute to the formation of these points (17).

1.3.10. Compression of a nerve root.

Compression or irritation of a nerve root can cause sensitization of the corresponding spinal segment and lead to the development of PGMs in the muscles innervated by that nerve root. This may occur due to herniated discs, spinal stenosis or other neurological conditions (17).

1.3.11. Chronic muscular imbalance.

Lack of physical activity can lead to weakening of dynamic muscles, making them more prone to developing PGMs. Inactivity can also contribute to poor posture and muscle imbalances. On the other hand, muscles that are inactive or not used properly can become weak and less efficient, which can lead to compensation by other muscles and the formation of PGMs. Conversely, if the muscles that work to maintain posture become excessively tight and stiff, especially if they are subjected to continuous stress or poor posture, it contributes to the formation of PGMs (17).

Myofascial pain triggers can also become long-lasting factors if not adequately addressed. Accurate identification and correction of these factors are critical to the effective management of myofascial pain and to prevent recurrence. Addressing not only the current pain, but also the underlying causes, can help eliminate pain and prevent its return.

Maintenance factors
Advanced age
Posture (including at work)
Obesity
Anorexia
Scar tissue (post-surgical)
Sports, leisure, habits
Stress and tension patterns
Metabolic disorders
Disease or disorder
Vitamin deficiencies
Congenital (bone) anomalies
Muscle fiber type
Direction / orientation of muscle fibers
Muscle shape / morphology (fusiform, etc.)
Psychological factors
Chronicity of trigger points

Table 1. Summary of maintenance factors at PGM points (18).

1.4. Symptoms and physical findings of trigger points.

To understand the origin of myofascial pain, it is essential to know two key concepts, muscle tension and trigger points. Muscle tension arises from the combination of two different factors, viscoelastic tone and contractile activity. Viscoelastic tone can be divided into viscoelastic stiffness and elastic stiffness. Elastic stiffness is related to motion, whereas viscoelastic stiffness is velocity-dependent. Contractile activity is classified into three types: contracture, electrogenic spasm (of pathological origin) and electrogenic stiffness. Contracture does not generate electromyographic activity and originates within the muscle fibers. Electrogenic spasm is a pathological and involuntary muscle contraction initiated in the alpha motor neurons and the motor plate. Electrogenic rigidity, on the other hand, refers to muscle tension resulting from contraction in people who are not relaxed (14).

Active PGs cause pain that the patient can identify when pressed, while latent PGs can increase muscle tension and cause shortening without spontaneous pain. Both types of PGs can generate significant motor dysfunction. Active PGs can induce satellite PGs in other muscles, and by treating the key PG, the satellite is often inactivated as well. PGs are commonly activated by muscle overload, whether acute, maintained or repetitive, or by holding the muscle in a shortened position. They can also be activated by nerve compression, disrupting communication between neurons and motor plates (1, 19).

Patients with active PGs often experience diffuse pain in muscles and joints, and the pain may radiate to a distance from the PG. The pain is referred in muscle-specific patterns and sometimes presents as numbness or paresthesia. In addition to pain, PGs can cause alterations in autonomic functions such as excessive sweating and balance problems, as well as muscle weakness and spasm. These dysfunctions can lead to decreased functional capacity and motor coordination (20, 21). Pain associated with PGs can disrupt sleep, intensifying pain sensitivity the next day. Holding the muscle in a shortened position or under pressure during sleep may increase pain and affect the quality of rest (22).

As for physical findings in a muscle affected by a PG, pain increases with stretching, and a decrease in muscle strength and endurance is also observed. PGs are identified as painful nodules in palpable tight bands within the muscles. The more active the PGs, the more severe the restriction in range of motion and increased muscle tension (1, 19).

On palpation of a superficial muscle, a nodule can be detected in the tense band, extending from the nodule to the muscle insertions. This sign may reduce or disappear after effective inactivation of the PG. Palpation reveals an extremely tender nodule within the taut band. The pain response may vary with small changes in applied pressure. For recognition, applying pressure to a PG may elicit a referred pain pattern that the patient may recognize as familiar, indicating that the PG is active. This is crucial for diagnosis. In addition to projected pain, PGs can cause hypersensitivity to pressure and dysesthesias (23).

Sudden palpation of a PG often causes a transient spasm in the muscle fibers. This spasm may be similar to that caused by the insertion of a needle. Active PGs reduce the range of passive motion due to pain. This limitation is more pronounced with passive stretching than with active muscle movement. Range of motion usually recovers once the PG is inactivated. When contracting a muscle with an active PG against a fixed resistance, pain intensifies, especially if the muscle is in a shortened position. Muscles with active PGs often show variable weakness between individuals and muscles (24, 25).

Electromyographic (EMG) studies show that these muscles fatigue faster and become exhausted earlier than normal muscles, often due to reflex inhibition caused by PG (26).

Symptoms of autonomic changes
Hypersalivation: increased saliva.
Epilora: abnormal overflow of tears running down the cheek
Conjunctivitis: eye reddening
Ptosis: eyelid puffiness Blurred vision
Increased nasal secrction.
Goose bumps

Summary of symptoms of autonomic changes (18).

Physical findings
Small nodules about the size of a pinhead.
Pea-sized nodules
Large lumps.
Several large packages side by side.
Soft spots submerged in taut bands of semi-hard muscle that are palpated like a rope.
Rope-like strips arranged side by side like partially cooked spaghetti.
The skin above a trigger point is often slightly warmer than the surrounding skin due to increased metabolic/autonomic activity.

Summary of physical findings (18).

2. CLINICAL EVALUATION OF MYOFASCIAL PAIN

2.1 Referred pain and tenderness.

Referred pain and hypersensitivity are key to identifying the muscles responsible for myofascial pain syndrome. Patients are often unaware of the trigger point (TP) in the muscle causing the pain, as the pain is often felt in areas away from the TP. Referred pain patterns are predictable and help localize the affected muscle. Myofascial pain is deep and continuous, although it may present as sharp stinging or stabbing. PG-referred pain patterns are usually directed toward the periphery of the body in 85% of cases, while only 10% of the patterns are local. The patterns are useful for localizing the PG, but relying solely on the location of the pain reported by the patient can lead to errors in most cases. For a correct evaluation, the use of trigger point charts is recommended. In addition, when PGs are more active, the pain is more widespread and intense (27).

In pain drawings, solid red areas represent essential areas of pain, while dotted areas show less common areas of pain. A black or white X indicates the frequent location of a PG, although they can be found anywhere in the affected muscle (1, 27).

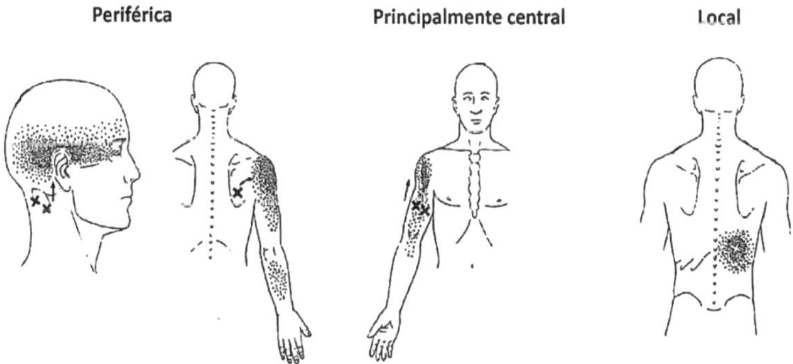

Figure 1. Directions in which PGMs can produce pain (1).

Pain pattern drawing is a useful tool for locating trigger points (TP) responsible for myofascial pain, as patients' verbal descriptions are often inaccurate. Blank body silhouettes are used for the patient or clinician to draw the pain areas, improving communication and diagnostic accuracy. This graphic recording is essential for comparing the patient's pain patterns with known patterns of individual muscles (1, 27).

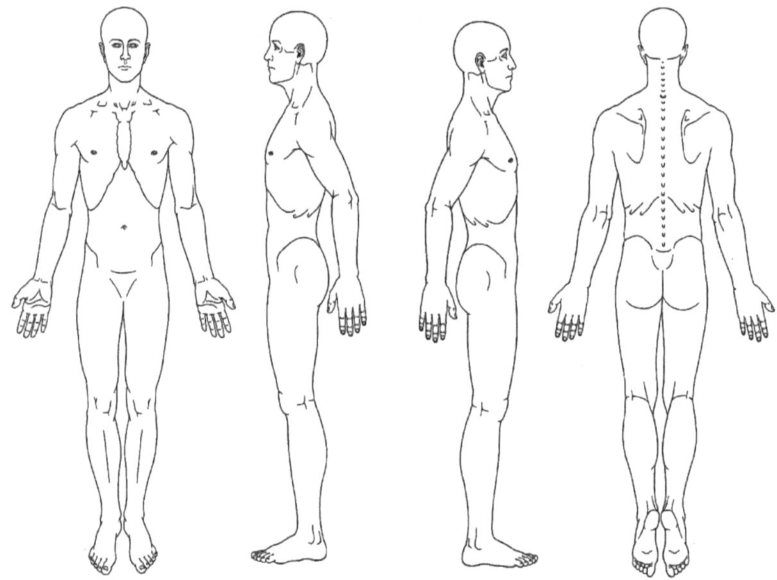

Figure 2. Body silhouette seen in frontal, left and right lateral and posterior views for marking the painful area or PGM (1).

The process consists of asking the patient to point to the painful area and having the clinician draw it on the silhouette. The patient then reviews the drawing to make it more accurate. Areas of more intense pain are marked with solid red, while areas of less frequent or less intense pain are dotted. For numbness or tingling, other colors may be used. Trigger points are marked with an X, and after treatment can be marked where it was applied (1, 27).

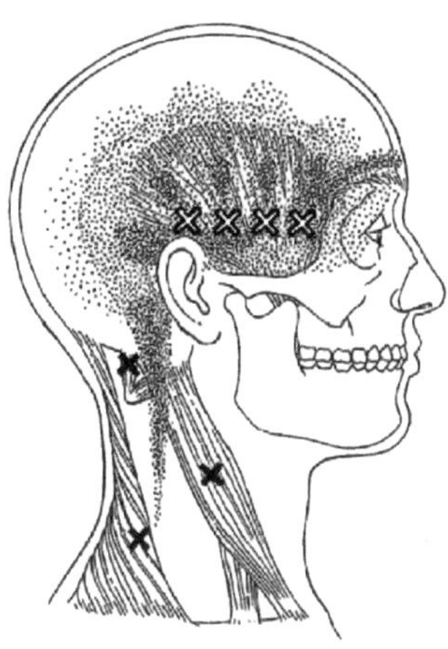

Pain pattern in common tension headache, caused by the superimposition of the referred patterns (dots) of MGP in temporal (white x), suboccipital (upper black x), ECOM (middle black x), and upper trapezius (lower black x) (1).

Recording these details helps monitor the evolution of the pain and provides a clearer picture of the source of the problem. In addition, comparing the patient's pattern with trigger point charts helps confirm that their pain is real and shared by other patients. This reinforces the patient's confidence and improves the relationship with the clinician. Interpretation of the initial pain patterns is key to determining whether the pain is coming from a myofascial trigger point (TP) from a single muscle or from several overlapping patterns. Myofascial patterns are rarely symmetrical and their extent may increase with PG activity. When several muscles refer pain to the same area, the area may be more painful and hyperaesthetic. For successful treatment, it is important to inactivate all involved PGs (1, 27).

The clinical history should include the evolution of the pain pattern, as a stable pattern suggests a more rapid resolution with appropriate treatment. If the pain has spread to multiple muscles, it is critical to eliminate the perpetuating factors for lasting relief. At follow-up visits, treatment success is measured by comparing previous pain patterns with current pain patterns. If the patient experiences the same pain after treatment, there may be unresolved perpetuating factors. If partial improvement is noted, the pain may have changed location, revealing other active PGs that need to be addressed. Keeping a detailed record of pain patterns is crucial for measuring progress and adjusting treatment (1, 27).

2.2 Methods of differential diagnosis of a trigger point.

Criteria for diagnosing myofascial pain syndrome vary among investigations, but the most common are (28, 29):

- The presence of a painful nodule in a tense and palpable muscle band.
- Reproduction of pain when pressing the myofascial trigger point. Myofascial pain syndrome is often confused with fibromyalgia.

According to the 1990 American College of Rheumatology (ACR) criteria, fibromyalgia is diagnosed based on (14, 30, 31):

- Chronic generalized pain above and below the waist, lasting more than three months.
- The presence of 11 of 18 established pain points. Recently, the 2010 criteria of the same institution have been published. Frequently, patients with fibromyalgia present with secondary myofascial trigger points. However, there is a clear clinical distinction between the two conditions, which is crucial, as the treatments are different.

2.3 Exploration, palpation and use of complementary tools in PGs.

Accurate identification of MMPs is key to diagnosing and treating myofascial pain. The following is a description of how to perform the exploration of MMPs and the associated diagnostic criteria (1, 32, 33).

The first step is to identify which muscles to explore based on the patient's range of motion limitations and pain patterns referred. The examiner can resist a movement to contract the suspected muscle and palpate it to confirm its location. It is essential that the patient is in a comfortable, relaxed position in a comfortable temperature environment. The muscle must be completely relaxed, since, if it is tense, it will be difficult to distinguish the tense bands associated with PGs from normal muscle fibers (1, 33).

Careful palpation is key to locating tight bands and nodules associated with PGs. There are three main palpation techniques (1, 32, 33):

- Flat palpation: It is used for superficial muscles, where it is palpated perpendicularly to the muscle fibers. It is a technique used to explore muscles that are only accessible from one side, such as the infraspinatus. This method makes it possible to detect tight bands within the muscle through the movement of the skin and the perception of changes in the muscle fibers. The procedure used is described in the figure below:

  Initiating palpation (Figure A), the examiner pushes the skin to one side so that it is mobilized over the muscle to be examined. This initial mobilization of the skin facilitates access to the underlying muscle fibers. Sliding the fingertip (Figure B), with the skin displaced, the fingertip slides transversely to the muscle fibers, allowing detection of the taut bands. These bands are felt as chordal structures rolling under the finger. The texture of these taut bands is firmer than that of normal muscle fibers. Finishing the movement (Figure C), at the end of the sliding across the muscle fibers, the skin is pushed to the other side, thus completing the palpation path. This maneuver not only makes it possible to identify the tight bands, but also to locate the point where the greatest pain is concentrated on pressure, corresponding to the trigger point. When this technique is performed more vigorously and quickly, it is known as sudden palpation, which can intensify the perception of tight bands and their diagnosis.

- Pincer palpation: Used when the muscle can be grasped between the fingers, such as the sternocleidomastoid. The following is a description of the procedure used in the figure below: Pincer palpation (Figure A), the muscle fibers of the muscle in question are grasped between the thumb and triphalangeal fingers, forming a pincer that allows the tension within the muscle to be captured. The tight band and trigger point are in this area. Perception of the taut band (Figure B), by pressing and letting the muscle fibers roll between the fingers, the hardness of the taut band is felt. The change in angle of the distal phalanges creates a rocking motion that enhances sensitivity and discrimination, helping to detect the stiff texture of the taut band and any fine details. Escaping from the fingers (Figure C), the palpable edge of the taut band is defined when it escapes from between the fingertips, which can often elicit a local twitch response. This phenomenon is characteristic of active trigger points.

- Deep palpation: For deep muscles where the previous techniques are not feasible.

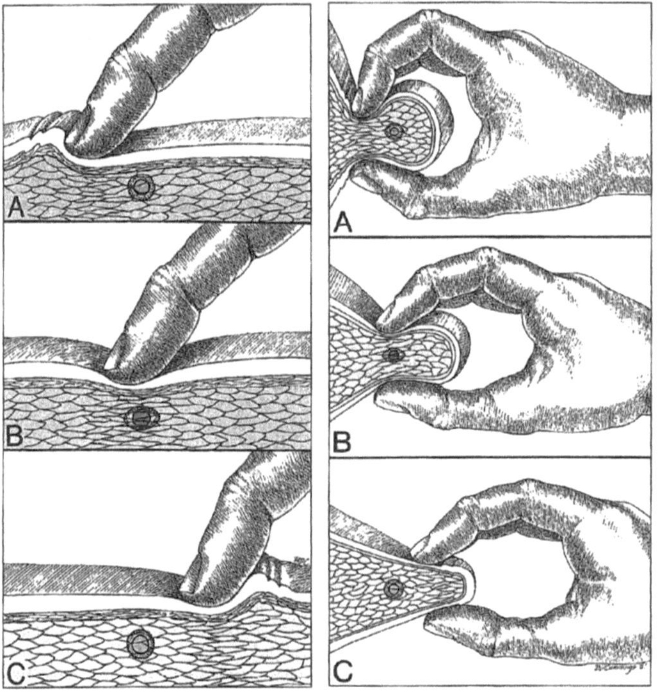

Figure 4. The image on the left shows the flat palpation of a tense band and its PGM. In the image on the right we find a pincer palpation of a tense band at the level of a PGM (1).

The examiner's fingernails should be short to avoid causing unnecessary pain to the patient, which could interfere with the correct identification of PGMs. Long nails may cause cutaneous pain to be mistaken for actual PG pain (1, 32, 33).

Although the use of dermometers (to measure skin conductance) has been suggested as a tool to detect PGMs, these devices are not sufficiently reliable. Further studies would be needed to evaluate their efficacy and reliability. The most reliable feature for diagnosing a PGM is the presence of exquisite pain on palpation of a nodule in a palpable tense band of muscle. If pressure on this nodule reproduces the patient's characteristic pain, the PGM is considered active. Other indicators, such as limitation in range of motion and local spasm response, also support the diagnosis (1, 32, 33).

PGMs can be difficult to detect, especially in deep muscles, and excessive pressure can trigger an exaggerated response in the patient, known as the "jump sign". To obtain a quantitative assessment of pain on pressure, an algometer can be used (1, 32, 33).

Currently, there are no widely accepted laboratory tests or imaging techniques to diagnose trigger points (TP). Diagnosis of myofascial pain syndrome remains predominantly clinical, although tools have recently been developed to help confirm the presence of PGs, with needle electromyography and ultrasonography being particularly promising for clinical use.

- Needle electromyography: This was initially explored in 1957 and was later found to detect electromyographic activity specific to myofascial PGs. Animal and human studies have confirmed the presence of characteristic activity, such as motor plate "noise" and high-voltage spikes, which are indicative of, but not exclusive to, PGs. Surface electromyography shows how PGs affect normal muscle function, increasing reactivity, delaying relaxation and causing increased fatigue. Recent research has used computer analysis to study how PGs influence muscle activity, revealing that they can affect motor function locally and in related muscles via the central nervous system. It has been observed that PGs can cause spasm in referred muscles and that some muscles tend to develop PGs in response to spasm in other muscles. This suggests a complex interaction between PG-affected muscles and their influence on the activity of other muscles. In addition, the presence of PGs may induce an abnormal motor reaction in nearby muscles. Finally, the ability of PGs to cause inhibition in muscle function can significantly alter normal muscle performance, and restoration of normal patterns may require reeducation of the affected muscle. These phenomena suggest that motor dysfunction caused by PGs is as complex as sensory dysfunction and deserves further investigation (25, 34, 35).

- Ultrasonography: It was first used by Michael Margolis to visualize the PG response. This technique can complement electromyographic recordings and has potential to be an effective diagnostic tool for PGs, although its application requires skill in palpation or insertion of a needle into the PG to elicit the expected response. The use of a 12.5 MHz transducer over a muscle band has shown a focused hypoechoic zone of 0.16 ± 0.11 cm^2, which has previously been identified as a myofascial trigger point. This zone does not appear in healthy muscle tissue or around other trigger points. Another study performed with a 7-12 MHz transducer on the anterior rectus also revealed changes in echogenicity in areas previously associated with myofascial trigger points. When using an ultrasound with a 5-12 MHz transducer, a higher frequency of local contractile response was observed when stimulating a trigger point, compared to clinical observation. This contraction was associated with a better response to treatment. However, in this study, no imaging abnormalities were found to correspond to myofascial trigger points, something that also occurred in another study with few patients. The cost of ultrasonography equipment has decreased considerably, while the quality of the images has improved. In our center, we have found hypoechoic areas with similar characteristics to those described by other authors that correlate clinically with myofascial trigger points. However, when interpreting these studies it is important to consider variables such as the characteristics of the equipment, the transducer, the operator's training, the patient's evolution time and the previous use of infiltrations (36, 37, 38, 39).
- Elastography, ultrasound and MRI: The use of imaging techniques such as elastography, ultrasound and MRI has allowed a more accurate assessment of myofascial trigger points (MTrPs). These tools help identify structural and functional changes in muscle tissue that are not always evident by traditional physical examination.

- Elastography has been shown to be effective in detecting increased muscle stiffness in areas affected by MMPs. Both ultrasound elastography and magnetic resonance elastography can identify and quantify the characteristic tight bands of PGMs, differentiating them from healthy tissue. These techniques allow a noninvasive and detailed assessment of changes in muscle elasticity, which facilitates the diagnosis and follow-up of patients (40, 41, 42).
- Ultrasound is another key tool in the evaluation of MMPs, especially to detect alterations in the structure and echogenicity of muscle tissue. Ultrasound imaging makes it possible to observe differences in muscle texture, such as hyperechogenic areas, which correspond to the areas where PGMs are located. In addition, its ability to visualize the tissue in real time makes it useful for guiding therapeutic interventions (43, 44, 45).
- On the other hand, magnetic resonance imaging (MRI) offers a deeper and more detailed view of the muscles affected by MMPs. It makes it possible to identify not only structural changes in the muscle, but also to evaluate the surrounding tissue, which is particularly useful in deeper or complex muscle areas. MRI complements ultrasound by providing higher resolution images for accurate diagnosis of PGMs (46, 47, 48).

Overall, these imaging technologies have proven to be valuable tools for improving the diagnosis and treatment of myofascial trigger points, providing objective information about alterations in muscle tissue structure and function. This facilitates a more accurate approach to treatment planning in patients with myofascial pain.

- Algometry: Measures pain sensitivity using pressure or electrical stimulation. Three types of information it provides have been identified (23, 49, 50).

- Local pain threshold: The pressure required for pain to be initiated at a specific point.
- Referred pain threshold: The pressure that causes pain in areas distant from the point of application.
- Pain tolerance: The maximum pressure the patient can withstand before the pain becomes intolerable.

The spring algometer, designed in 1986 and widely used since then, measures these thresholds by applying pressure to the skin using a calibrated circular tip. The measurement is made in Kg or Newtons, and the accuracy depends on the diameter of the algometer tip. This instrument is useful for comparing pain sensitivity before and after treatments. However, it has limitations such as, it does not determine the cause of the pain, which can be myofascial, fibromyalgia, bursitis, etc. The measurement can be affected by tissue thickness and muscle sensitivity. The technique requires dexterity and correct localization of the point of maximum sensitivity. Recent research has shown that algometry may not clearly distinguish between active and latent trigger points, and that results may vary depending on the pressure applied. Although useful for research and clinical purposes, it should be interpreted with caution (23, 49, 50).

- Thermography: Using infrared radiometry or liquid crystal films, it measures changes in skin temperature. Electronic thermography is more accurate and convenient, showing thermal variations that can indicate problems such as myofascial trigger points. However, a thermal change does not always indicate a trigger point, as it may be caused by other conditions such as radiculopathy or local inflammation. Studies have found that the skin temperature over a trigger point may be higher, but this does not always translate into accurate trigger point detection. Studies also show that active trigger points can cause hyperthermia in the skin, while mechanical stimulation can cause "reflex" hypothermia. Thermography can identify hot areas, but it can also have false positives and negatives. Combining thermography with other methods, such as palpation and algometric measurement, improves the accuracy of trigger point identification. However, interpretation of the results should be done with caution and complemented with other diagnostic evaluations (51, 52, 53, 54).

So far, the literature has not addressed some key questions about the thermal changes associated with trigger points (TP). Since many acupuncturists employ devices to measure skin resistance to identify the optimal place to insert the needle and treat a PG or sore spot, it would be of great interest to conduct a blinded study to investigate the region of a hot spot and look for points of low resistance. It would be useful to determine how often these low resistance points coincide with hot spots and whether these points have a PG (active or latent) nearby. PG identification should be based on accurate diagnostic criteria applied by evaluators with high interexaminer reliability. Furthermore, since several studies have shown that PG dysfunction is influenced by sympathetic nervous system activity, investigating how PGs affect sympathetic control of cutaneous perfusion could enrich our understanding of the relationship between myofascial PGs and the autonomic nervous system.

3. FUNDAMENTALS OF DRY NEEDLING (PS)

Anatomical considerations for PS.

Dry needling involves certain risks to various anatomical structures, such as organs, nerves and blood vessels. Therefore, it is essential that practitioners have a solid anatomical knowledge, both theoretical and practical, to minimize complications (1, 32, 55, 56).

- Pleura and lungs: Pneumothorax is a serious, although rare, complication of PS. It can be avoided if the physiotherapist applies anatomical knowledge correctly. It is essential to avoid directing the needle into the lungs or intercostal space. Use the pincer palpation technique to puncture muscles such as the trapezius, pectoralis and latissimus dorsi, or direct the needle into bony structures, such as ribs or scapula, to prevent access to the pleura.
- Blood vessels: It is crucial to identify and avoid blood vessels. Knowledge of vascular anatomy allows the clinician to avoid puncturing superficial veins by inspection and palpation of arteries by pulse. Apply pressure to ensure hemostasis after needle withdrawal, especially in patients with thrombocytopenia.
- Nerves: Needle insertion near nerves requires caution to avoid injury. If the patient experiences sharp, electric pain, the needle may have touched a nerve. The area near the spinal cord and the suboccipital area should be avoided due to the risks of affecting the brainstem.
- Organs: The physical therapist should be aware of the location of internal organs to avoid punctures. For example, there is a risk when puncturing the psoas major or quadratus lumborum muscles due to the proximity to the kidney, or when approaching the abdominal muscles near the peritoneal organs.
- Joints: It is important to avoid puncturing joints, joint capsules or bursae, as it can lead to infections in these sensitive structures.

- Prostheses and implanted devices: Avoid puncturing near prostheses (limbs, internal and external fixations) or implanted devices (pacemakers, breast or buttock implants, etc.) to prevent infection and damage to the devices.
- Pathological areas: It is also crucial to avoid areas affected by acute inflammations, infections, varicose veins, cysts, tumors or skin lesions to avoid further complications.

With this knowledge, clinicians can minimize the risks associated with PS by applying appropriate techniques and taking the necessary precautions.

Therapeutic effectiveness and indications in dry needling.

3.1.1 Therapeutic effectiveness.

The key to effective dry needling (DP) is accurate diagnosis of myofascial trigger points (MTrPs) and myofascial pain syndrome (MPS). Without proper diagnosis, SP can be unsafe and generate questionable results.

The first clinical trial in which SP was used to treat musculoskeletal pain was in 1941, although the term "dry needling" was not used until 1947. This study compared three groups of patients with low back pain, one receiving novocaine, one receiving saline and one receiving the puncture alone. Surprisingly, the results were similar in all groups, suggesting that the needle itself had a therapeutic effect. Since then, multiple studies have demonstrated the effectiveness of PS, similar to that of anesthetic infiltrations. Subsequent research, such as that of Hong in 1994, confirmed that both PS and lidocaine infiltration are effective when eliciting local twitch responses (REL), although PS eliciting REL is more effective than infiltration without REL (57).

Despite the clinical evidence in favor of PS for numerous conditions, such as myofascial pain, neck and low back pain, headaches, migraines and more, more research is needed. Systematic reviews indicate that PS is effective, but superiority to placebo has not yet been demonstrated, posing challenges in the design of double-blind, controlled studies. Although placebo needles exist, they can generate physiological stimulation that complicates assessment of their true placebo effect. In an effort to address these challenges, some recent studies have applied treatments under anesthesia to ensure adequate masking, with promising results. Current evidence increasingly supports the use of PS, especially for immediate pain relief in patients with MDS, although further research is recommended (58, 59, 60).

3.1.2 Indications for dry needling.

Indications for dry needling (DP) refer to conditions in which this technique has been shown to be effective or its use is suggested. Among the main indications are (58, 59, 60).

- Myofascial pain: Pain caused by the presence of myofascial trigger points (MTrPs) in muscles.
- Shoulder pain: Including pain in hemiparesis, chronic subacromial syndrome (impingement), and adhesive capsulitis.
- Chronic lumbar and cervical pain: Associated with cervical or lumbar radiculopathies and whiplash syndrome.
- Headaches and migraines: For the treatment of tension headaches and chronic migraines.
- Post-surgical pain: In cases of chronic postoperative pain in the thorax or knees.
- Carpal tunnel syndrome and other nerve entrapments.
- Tendinopathies: Pain caused by inflammation or degeneration of tendons.
- Plantar fasciitis: Chronic pain in the sole of the foot.
- Chronic pelvic pain: Associated with muscular conditions.
- Piriformis syndrome and sciatica: radiating pain in the leg.
- Muscle spasticity: In patients with cerebral palsy or incomplete spinal cord injury.
- Phantom limb pain: In post-amputation patients.
- Temporomandibular dysfunction: Pain and dysfunction in the jaw joint.

These indications are based on clinical studies and observations on the ability of dry needling to deactivate PGMs and reduce pain in various areas of the body.

Precautions in PS.

The hazards associated with dry needling (DP) are rare and their likelihood is low, especially if proper precautions are taken. However, it is essential that the physical therapist assess the risks versus the benefits of the technique, using his or her clinical judgment on a case-by-case basis. Non-invasive treatment should be considered to achieve the desired goals. The following are precautions to be taken into account (61, 62, 63).

3.1.3 Pain.

Pain is one of the most common adverse effects during trigger point treatment using PS. This pain can be severe when a local spasm response is elicited upon needle insertion. Although one study indicates a mean visual analog scale (VAS) pain of 5.25, clinical experience suggests that pain can often exceed 7 points. Post puncture pain can be significant, but is usually temporary and subsides within a few hours. A distinction should be made between post-puncture pain and referred pain that the patient was already experiencing. In research, it has been found that almost all patients undergoing PS report some post-puncture pain, although this is usually considered more tolerable compared to the previous pain. Most of these symptoms are transient and do not usually cause serious complications (61, 62, 63).

3.1.4 Problems with needles

The use of needles in PS can lead to complications such as bending, jamming, breaking or getting lost. These problems are relatively common, but usually have minor consequences. Broken or forgotten needles are less common, although they can have serious consequences. To prevent needles from getting stuck or bent, it is crucial that the physical therapist maintains good control and has good technique. In rare cases, there may be incidents of forgotten needles in the patient, which could carry risks, so it is advisable to keep an accurate count of the needles used (61, 62, 63).

3.1.5 Pneumothorax.

Pneumothorax is a serious but rare complication that can arise from acupuncture or PS. It consists of the accumulation of air in the pleural cavity, which can lead to lung collapse. Although it is a potential risk, its occurrence is rare and can usually be prevented by proper anatomical knowledge and careful needling techniques. It is advisable to avoid performing deep punctures on both sides of the chest in the same session and to consider the use of ultrasound or alternative manual techniques if there are doubts about the safe performance of PS. Continuous training and attention to technique are essential to minimize these risks (61, 62, 63).

3.1.6 Vascular lesions in PS.

Dry needling is a technique that, although effective for the treatment of various muscular conditions, carries the risk of causing vascular injury. Understanding the anatomy of the vascular system is essential to avoid complications. At the start of the procedure, the physical therapist should be aware of the location of the major vessels and, as far as possible, palpate the pulses. However, some peripheral vessels are difficult to identify, which can complicate the technique. When a needle punctures a blood vessel, the patient usually feels a prick or stinging sensation, different from puncturing muscle tissue. Although these injuries may go unnoticed, they can result in serious bleeding. The most common complications include bleeding and hematoma formation. Although these are considered minor adverse effects, their implications can be significant. It is critical to distinguish between bleeding that occurs in muscle tissue and superficial bleeding that affects vessels at the cutaneous and subcutaneous level. The former can lead to alterations in local pH, affecting muscle function and causing additional discomfort. To manage any bleeding that arises, the therapist should apply firm pressure over the puncture site, maintaining it for at least 3 to 10 minutes, especially if a vessel is suspected to have been punctured (61, 62, 63, 64, 65).

Patients with vascular disease or those receiving anticoagulant therapy should be monitored with particular attention, as they are more prone to complications. In these cases, less invasive techniques should be adopted and extreme precautions should be taken, maintaining adequate hemostatic pressure after the procedure. Although severe complications, such as pseudoaneurysms or compartment syndromes, are rare, detailed anatomical knowledge and careful application of techniques can help prevent these situations (61, 62, 63, 64, 65).

3.1.7 Nerve lesions in PS for the peripheral nervous system (PNS).

In addition to vascular injuries, nerve injuries represent a significant risk in dry needling. To avoid these complications, it is vital that the physical therapist has a clear understanding of the anatomy and peripheral nerve pathways. Some areas of risk include muscles close to nerve structures, such as the piriformis and iliopsoas. One of the key precautions is not to insert the needle all the way to the handle, as the part closest to the skin is the most fragile and can cause complications if it gets close to a nerve. Needle insertion should be done slowly and carefully, watching for any signs the patient may provide. If the patient reports an electrical or stabbing sensation, this may indicate that a nerve has been pinched. In such a case, it is crucial to withdraw the needle and change the direction of insertion (61, 62, 63, 64, 65).

The use of ultrasound may be particularly beneficial in identifying nerve structures and minimizing the risk of accidental punctures. Although serious complications from nerve puncture are rare, cases of neuroparalysis and other adverse reactions have been documented. Studies have shown that among treated patients, mild reactions, such as tingling and paresthesia, have been reported. Fortunately, most of these cases are manageable, and patients tend to recover without significant complications. To mitigate the risk of nerve injury, it is crucial that the physical therapist exercise caution, adjusting his or her technique according to the sensations reported by the patient during the procedure (61, 62, 63, 64, 65).

3.1.8 Nerve injuries in PS for the central nervous system (CNS).

Nerve injuries represent one of the most critical complications in the practice of dry needling, especially when dealing with areas close to the central nervous system. Protection of the spinal cord is essential, especially when working with the deep paravertebral musculature or in the cervical spine muscles. To minimize the risk of contact with the spinal cord during dry needling, several recommendations should be followed (61, 62, 63, 64, 65):

- Needle length: It is important to use needles of adequate length. Needles of 40 mm are recommended for the cervical and thoracic regions, and 50 mm for the lumbar and sacral regions.
- Angle of insertion: When puncturing the deep paravertebral musculature, the needle should be inserted between 1 cm and 1.5 cm from the line of the spinous processes, with a craniocaudal inclination of approximately 10° to 15° along the spine. This prevents the needle from passing through the intervertebral spaces or the facet joints, reducing the risk of epidural or subdural hematomas.
- Bone reference: Contact with the vertebral lamina, which acts as a barrier in front of the spinal canal, should be sought. This helps to confirm that the different strata of the transverse spinous muscles have been crossed. If the needle is introduced beyond the expected distances from the bone, the direction of the puncture should be adjusted.
- Precautions in the suboccipital triangle: In this area, bounded by the posterior greater rectus abdominis, superior oblique and inferior oblique muscles, it is vital to be especially careful. When working in this area or above the level of C2, the vertebral artery is exposed and unprotected.
- Patient sensations: During needle insertion, slow entry is crucial. The patient should be informed to report if he/she feels an electrical sensation, which may indicate nerve contact.

Although serious adverse reactions due to contact with the central nervous system are rare, there are documented cases. A study by Ernst et al. reported six adverse events, including (66, 67):

- Cervical spinal cord injury, resulting in a permanent deficit.
- Subarachnoid hemorrhage with no information on treatment or recovery.

- Epidural hematoma that recovered completely.
- Three cases related to broken needle fragments causing complications that were resolved surgically.
- Peuker et al. reviewed the literature and found ten cases of spinal cord or nerve root injuries, as well as cases of arachnoiditis and subarachnoid hemorrhages during sessions of acupuncture. In their review, no vertebral artery injuries were found.

The chances of causing central nervous system injury are remote if safety recommendations are followed, which include slow needle entry and proper choice of needle length, as well as maintaining suggested angles of inclination and avoiding puncture above C2.

3.1.9 Visceral lesions in PS.

The most common visceral injury in dry needling is pneumothorax. Some muscles are close to abdominal viscera, which may cause unintentional injuries when treating muscles such as the psoas, quadratus lumborum or abdominal musculature. Although these events are rare, some have been documented as (65, 66, 67):

- A needle fragment lodged in the kidney.
- A retroperitoneal hematoma.
- A renal complication following urinary bladder injury.
- A case of pancreatitis due to direct puncture.

In addition to the risks associated with pneumothorax, there is the potential for more serious injury, such as cardiac tamponade. The latter involves the accumulation of blood or fluid in the space between the myocardium and the pericardium, which can compromise cardiac function and be fatal if action is not taken quickly. In some cases, the needle has passed through the sternum due to a malformation known as sternal foramen, present in 5-8% of the population.

To avoid visceral complications, it is essential to have a good knowledge of the anatomy of the area and to adopt rigorous aseptic measures. Although there are few documented cases of significant visceral injury, it is essential to be aware of the risk of infection, which is the most common complication in this setting.

3.1.10 Infections.

The risk of infection in dry needling is considerable for both the patient and the physical therapist in the event of an accidental puncture with a used needle. Although the risk of infection is generally low, it is crucial to follow proper protocols to minimize this risk.

Considering the risk of infection to the patient when inserting a needle into the body, there is an inherent risk of infection. It is estimated that about 1,000 bacteria inhabit each square centimeter of skin, with more numerous bacteria in the underlying ducts and glands. However, these bacteria have little potential to cause infection, as illustrated in the work of Dann (68), who reported no infections after more than 5,000 injections without skin preparation. Wit et al (69). documented local infections in 0.014% of the 230,000 patients studied. In the review by Ernst et al. 38 serious infections were reported, especially septic arthritis and psoas abscesses, all of which were satisfactorily treated. Zhang et al (70). reported cases of bacterial and viral infections, emphasizing that these are generally due to bad practices, such as the use of reused and poorly sterilized needles.

To prevent infections in the physical therapist due to accidental punctures, should be considered (66, 67, 68):

- Careful needle handling: Avoid reinserting the needle into the guide tube in an unsafe manner and be careful when performing clamp punctures.
- Safe disposal: Take care when disposing of needles in specific containers to avoid accidental punctures.

By following these guidelines, the risk of complications associated with dry needling can be significantly reduced for both the patient and the physical therapist.

To minimize the risk of infection, the following precautions should be taken (69, 70, 71):

- Hand washing: Before performing the puncture, it is crucial to wash hands thoroughly with soap and water or a hydroalcoholic solution, even if gloves are used.
- Disinfection of the area: Although there is no consensus on its efficacy, it is recommended to clean the puncture site with 70° alcohol to reduce the number of germs.
- Use of sterile needles: Needles should be sterile and for single use only. They should never be reused for different treatments, even for the same patient.
- Careful handling of the needle: Handle the needle from the handle and avoid touching the part that will come into contact with the patient, unless absolutely necessary.
- Proper disposal of needles: Needles should be deposited in a specific container for biocontaminated material and replaced when the indicated limit is reached.
- Use of gloves: The use of latex or nitrile gloves is recommended, as they reduce the possibility of contagion in case of accidental puncture.

3.1.11 Vegetative reactions.

Vegetative reactions are common after puncture and may include vasovagal syncope, which is the most common adverse effect. They occur most frequently when the patient is in an upright position. Other symptoms include dizziness, sweating, tachycardia, and changes in blood pressure. Performing the puncture in the decubitus position is essential to prevent syncope and minimize the risk of injury in case of fainting (70, 71).

3.1.12 Puncture in pregnancy.

Caution should be exercised when performing punctures in pregnant women due to the possibility of miscarriage and misperceptions of causality by the patient or family members. It is recommended to avoid invasive techniques and opt for less aggressive methods, unless necessary. There is no scientific evidence to support the existence of "forbidden points" in acupuncture that could induce abortion. However, the risks should be considered (69, 70, 71).

3.1.13 Needle accidents in PS.

In the practice of PS, various needle accidents can occur, and it is crucial to know how to handle them properly. The most common accidents and their respective handling maneuvers are described below (66, 67, 68, 69):

- Bent needle: The needle may bend if the patient performs an intense muscular contraction while the needle is inserted. The needle should be withdrawn down to the subcutaneous tissue. Check if the needle is bent, if so, dispose of it properly to avoid risks of unwanted insertion or breakage.
- Stuck needle: The needle may get stuck in the skin or muscle. For its management we should ask the patient to relax as much as possible, try to extract the needle every 10-15 seconds, gently tap the skin around the needle and scrape the handle of the needle with the fingernail and try to extract it slowly. If the needle is very fixed, try to pinch the skin fold where it is inserted, to free it a little more and then try to pull it out. If the needle is stuck due to muscle spasm, two superficial needles can be inserted on both sides to help release the spasm.
- Blunt needle: Discard the needle immediately, as it may increase pain during manipulation.
- Broken needle: Inform the patient to remain calm to prevent the needle from penetrating deeper. Mark a circle around the insertion site for reference. If a piece of needle is exposed, attempt to remove it with forceps. If no fragments are exposed, apply pressure to the surrounding skin to facilitate removal with forceps. If it cannot be removed in consultation, specialized medical attention will be required for surgical removal.
- Important considerations:
    - Needle quality: Always use needles with the European Community quality seal.
    - Insertion length: Always keep a margin of 0.5 cm to 1 cm of needle outside the skin to facilitate its removal in case of emergency.

These accidents can be serious, so it is essential that physical therapists practicing dry needling are well informed and prepared to handle them properly.

3.2 Contraindications in PS.

It is essential to know the absolute and relative contraindications, as well as the special precautions in the practice of PS. A complete evaluation of the patient should be performed to detect possible risks and diseases that may influence the treatment. PS should be avoided in the following situations (72, 73, 74, 75):

- Absolute contraindications:
  - Needle phobia.
  - Patient refusal due to fear or beliefs.
  - Inability to give consent (cognitive, communication or age-related problems).
  - Medical emergencies or acute conditions.
  - Areas with lymphedema, due to increased risk of infection.
  - Other medical reasons that advise against PS.
- Relative contraindications

Once absolute contraindications have been ruled out, the clinician must assess the appropriateness of the treatment, considering the clinical history and the potential benefits versus risks. Some relative contraindications include:

- Tendency to hemorrhage: Patients with hemophilia, thrombocytopenia or on anticoagulant therapy require special attention.
- Immune system compromise: Those with immunosuppressive diseases (HIV, cancer, etc.) or under immunosuppressive treatment are at higher risk of infection.
- Vascular diseases: They may predispose to hematomas, hemorrhages and infections.

- Diabetes: Affects the regenerative capacity and circulation, increasing the risk of infections and hindering healing.
- Pregnancy: Caution should be exercised, especially in the first trimester, due to potential risks.

- Other special precautions:
  - Children: Parental or guardian consent is required, and deep PS should be avoided in children under 13-15 years of age.
  - Weakened or fragile patients: They may not tolerate the treatment adequately.
  - Epilepsy: Patients should not be left unsupervised while the needles are in place.
  - Psychological state: Anxiety or stress may interfere with tolerance to treatment.
  - Allergies: Especially to metals in needles (nickel, chromium) or latex in gloves.
  - Use of medications: Those that may affect the patient's immune system, coagulation or emotional stability should be taken into account.

In case of doubt about the patient's suitability, the treatment should be reconsidered or discarded to avoid risks.

Safety conditions.

Dry needling (SP) is an invasive procedure used in physical therapy and other disciplines to treat pain and muscle dysfunction. However, as a treatment involving the insertion of needles into tissues, it carries risks that are different from those associated with noninvasive therapies. Therefore, this section will focus on the safety of dry needling, addressing the considerations necessary to ensure the health of both patients and healthcare professionals involved in its application. SP can be divided into two categories: superficial dry needling (SDP) and trigger point dry needling (TPD). Each of these techniques has its own particularities and associated risks. It is essential that both healthcare professionals and patients understand the nature of these risks. According to the World Health Organization (WHO), the well-being of the patient is the highest priority, but it is also crucial to care for the health and safety of the practitioners and others who may be involved in the treatment (76, 77, 78).

The risks associated with PSPG are significant and can include hematoma, pneumothorax, infection, internal tissue injury and bleeding. The term "adverse effect" (AE) is used to describe any negative effect that may arise from a treatment, regardless of its severity. The classification of AEs can range from mild, which are brief and reversible, to severe, which may require hospitalization or result in significant disabilities or even death of the patient. Although the scientific literature still lacks comprehensive studies on PSPG-specific AEs, clinical experience suggests that serious adverse effects are infrequent. However, further research is essential to quantify these risks and provide a sound basis for informed patient consent (76, 77, 78).

Several studies have investigated the safety of acupuncture and have found that, although there are adverse effects, the incidence of serious events is low. For example, one study that analyzed 32,000 treatments performed by British physiotherapists and physicians found that most adverse effects were of low severity and often reversible. Other studies have shown a similar frequency of adverse effects in large cohorts of patients receiving acupuncture treatment, with bleeding and pain at the puncture site being the most common adverse effects (76, 77, 78).

However, it is important for healthcare professionals to be aware of the potential risks and adverse effects associated with any technique they use, including PSPG. Ongoing training and education on anatomy and needling techniques are crucial to minimize the risk of complications. Physical therapists should be proactive in identifying potential adverse effects and educating the patient about these risks. This includes the importance of informed consent, where patients should be informed not only about the benefits of treatment, but also about potential adverse effects (76, 77, 78).

3.2.1 Hand hygiene.

Dry needling (D&C) is an invasive procedure that carries certain risks, including the risk of healthcare-associated infections. The causative agents of these infections are diverse and include bacteria such as Staphylococcus and E. coli, viruses such as hepatitis B and C, human immunodeficiency virus (HIV), fungi such as Candida albicans, protozoa such as toxoplasma and prions that can cause diseases such as Creutzfeldt-Jakob disease (79).

To better understand the transmission of infectious diseases, it is useful to refer to the concept of the chain of infection, which is made up of six essential elements: an infectious agent, a reservoir (the area where the agent is found), an exit gate (the means by which the agent leaves the infected), a means of transmission, an entry gate (the way in which the agent enters the new host) and, finally, a susceptible host that can be infected. This model is fundamental for developing effective prevention strategies (79,80).

Standard precautions, developed and published by the Centers for Disease Control and Prevention, are a set of clinical guidelines designed to prevent the transmission of infectious agents. Their main objective is to interrupt the chain of infection by focusing on the mode of transmission, the gateway of entry and the susceptible host. These precautions require healthcare professionals to assume that any person can potentially be infected or colonized by microorganisms that can be transmitted in the healthcare setting. Therefore, they should apply a series of work practices to minimize the risk of contamination. These practices include critical aspects such as hand hygiene, glove use, proper skin preparation, safe handling of needles and medical waste, and prevention of needlestick injuries (80).

Hand hygiene is considered the most important intervention to prevent the transmission of infections. Recommendations related to this practice have been classified into three categories, according to the level of evidence supporting them (81):

- Category I refers to solid evidence supported by experimental, clinical or epidemiological studies.
- Category II includes results suggestive of clinical or epidemiological studies.
- Category III is based on the recommendations of healthcare experts based on their experience.

To carry out effective hand hygiene, it is essential that the nails are short and perfectly manicured. False nails, nail extensors and the use of varnish or nail polish should be avoided. In addition, it is advisable to remove any type of jewelry or costume jewelry from the hands and wrists, except for the wedding ring, and the sleeves of shirts should be short or rolled up. Hand decontamination is preferably performed with a suitable soap and water, although if the hands are visibly clean of contaminants, an appropriate gel or alcohol solution may be used. Hand decontamination is recommended in several specific situations, such as when hands are visibly soiled, before and after each patient contact, at the beginning and end of each work shift, after removing gloves, when leaving a contaminated area, after using soiled equipment or materials, after performing personal body functions, and before handling food (80, 81).

Attention to hand decontamination technique is crucial because, despite its apparent simplicity, incorrect techniques are commonly applied by health care professionals . Hand washing with conventional soap can remove visible soil, but is often less effective in preventing microorganism activity. On the other hand, alcoholic handwashing solutions have been shown to be more effective in this regard. Antimicrobial soaps prove to be more effective than conventional soaps, achieving a statistically significant reduction in microbial activity. However, the use of alcohol in gels is superior to antimicrobial or mild non-alcoholic soaps (82, 83)

Recommendations for proper hand washing with soap are as follows: first, wet hands with water; then apply an adequate amount of soap as directed by the manufacturer; rub hands vigorously for at least 15 seconds, making sure to cover all hand and finger surfaces; rinse hands with water; dry with a good quality disposable paper towel; use the towel to turn off the faucet and dispose of it in a bucket with a pedal; and avoid using hot water, as it can increase skin dryness and contribute to dermatitis (82, 83).

Alternatively, hands can be decontaminated with an alcohol solution or hand gel, as long as they are visibly clean. However, it is important to note that organic material can inactivate these solutions, so if the hands are soiled, they should be washed beforehand. It is recommended that the alcohol solution have a concentration of approximately 70% isopropanol, ethanol or n-propanol, as higher concentrations may increase the risk of dryness and dermatitis. It is suggested that hands be washed with soap every 5-10 applications of alcoholic gel to reconstitute the skin emollients (82, 83).

Given that healthcare professionals may perform up to 30 hand washes in a single work shift, there is a significant risk of skin irritation and dermatitis. Irritant dermatitis is a non-immunologic inflammatory response of the skin to an external agent, which can make the skin more susceptible to colonization by microorganisms. Therefore, prevention and treatment of all forms of dermatitis are crucial for the safety of both patients and healthcare professionals. To prevent occupational dermatitis in the healthcare setting, it is recommended to follow the manufacturer's instructions on the use of hand hygiene products, choose products with a low irritant potential and use emollients whenever possible. It is also important to pay attention to feedback from professionals on the products they use, as well as to use appropriate hand lotions that help maintain hydration and restore skin lipids (79, 81).

3.2.2 Gloves.

The use of gloves is essential in dry needling because they prevent contact with blood and other body fluids, especially in view of the frequent risk of hemorrhage. Although some argue that gloves may affect touch sensitivity, their use is mandatory according to regulations, and they must be disposable after each use. In the case of latex allergies, nitrile gloves are preferred. In addition, after their removal, it is necessary to wash the hands to avoid bacterial proliferation. Disinfection of the patient's skin before puncture is generally not necessary if it is visibly clean, following WHO recommendations. However, in some countries the use of disinfectants, such as isopropyl alcohol, is required, especially in areas with a higher risk of moisture accumulation. For immunocompromised patients, more rigorous preparation with specific disinfectant solutions, such as 2% iodine in alcohol, is recommended. Needles and other medical waste should be disposed of according to local regulations, using special sharps containers. These should be easily accessible during the procedure, but out of reach of children, and should not be filled above the safety line to avoid accidents (82, 83, 84, 85).

Puncture wounds (LP) are a common risk for healthcare professionals. These injuries can transmit dangerous pathogens such as HIV and hepatitis B and C viruses. Although the risk is lower with solid filament needles, it is crucial to maintain proper hygiene and waste disposal practices . In the event of an LP, the wound should be washed immediately, the incident reported, and medical attention sought. To prevent these injuries, practitioners should monitor needle use and disposal carefully, avoid interruptions, and work under optimal conditions. In addition, they should be vaccinated against hepatitis A and B. Not only practitioners, but also patients and their families are at risk if needles are not properly disposed of, so it is essential to maintain a safe environment (82, 83, 84, 85).

3.2.3 Safety during the procedure.

Dry needling (DP) is an invasive procedure that may be associated with adverse effects. Patient education and good communication with the clinician are essential for safe and effective practice. Pain after dry needling, known as post-treatment discomfort (MTT), is common and can last from 1 to 4 days. This discomfort is more common with deep trigger point dry needling (DTP) and less likely with superficial dry needling (SD). Patients should be informed about these possible discomforts to avoid unnecessary concerns. It is important to communicate with the patient to adjust the treatment according to their tolerance. If the patient experiences persistent, sharp pain during needle insertion, the needle should be removed and repositioned to a nearby area. Sharp or electrical pain may indicate that the needle has touched a nerve or blood vessel, in which case it should be withdrawn immediately and pressure applied to control possible bleeding (78, 88).

Hematoma is a frequent adverse effect. To reduce its occurrence, it is essential to avoid puncturing blood vessels and to apply manual pressure after needle removal. In case of skin bleeding, pressure should be used and ice should be applied if necessary. Fainting may occur during treatment due to factors such as pain, stress or needle phobia. To prevent this, the patient should be treated in a lying position. Maintain constant communication and avoid aggressive techniques. If the patient shows signs of dizziness or sweating, remove the needle and consider elevating the legs (78, 88).

Although the risk of infection is low, it is important to follow strict hygiene protocols. The puncture site should be inspected before and after treatment to identify possible signs of infection (pain, redness, fever, etc.). In punctures close to the thorax, there is a low but potential risk of pneumothorax. If suspected, the patient should be taken to the emergency department. Some patients may experience fatigue or drowsiness after SP. They should be warned not to drive or operate machinery until these symptoms disappear (78, 88).

4. DRY NEEDLING TECHNIQUES

4.1 Classification and modalities of the PS.

Dry needling (DP) is a technique used to treat myofascial trigger points (MTrPs) and has different modalities. These can be classified according to several criteria, such as the tool used, the type of stimulation, the depth of needle insertion, the conceptual model on which the technique is based or the practitioner performing the technique. However, the most commonly used criterion is the depth of the needle in relation to the PGM. There are two broad categories: superficial dry needling (SDP) and deep dry needling (DDP). In PSS, the needle does not penetrate the PGM, while in PSP the needle penetrates the PGM. Regarding the modalities, the best known are:

For PSS is the Peter Baldry technique, in which the needle is inserted into the subcutaneous tissues without reaching the PGM. This technique proved effective in reducing pain and hyperalgesia associated with PGMs, even in deep muscles. It is characterized by leaving the needle in the skin for 30 seconds, and if pain persists, the insertion time can be extended or additional stimulation can be applied (56, 89, 90).

Another technique is Fu subcutaneous puncture, which requires specific needles and seeks to mobilize the needle in the subcutaneous tissue at a certain distance from the PGM. This movement is repeated several times, and the catheter used can be left inside the body for several hours (89, 90, 91, 92, 93).

Regarding PSP, Hong's rapid entry and exit technique, which seeks to provoke local spasm responses (REL) by rapidly inserting and withdrawing the needle from the PGM, stands out. RELs are an indicator of treatment efficacy, and the number of insertions depends on patient tolerance (89, 90, 91, 92, 93).

Another technique that can be found is Gunn's intramuscular stimulation. This diagnostic and therapeutic approach focuses on the treatment of chronic pain, suggesting that trigger points myofascial (PGM) are a consequence of radiculopathies or alterations of the nervous system.

It uses acupuncture needles inserted and manipulated with an injector, making rapid entries and exits and twists in both directions to elicit an endorphin release response (REL) or referred pain. If the pain does not disappear or increases, it is recommended to discontinue the technique (89, 90, 91, 92, 93).

The rapid entry and exit technique with rotation is the adaptation of the multiple insertion technique, designed to facilitate needle insertion without bending. The needle is rotated on insertion and withdrawal, and is further detailed in the corresponding chapter (89, 90, 91, 92, 93).

The needle twisting technique is proposed as a less aggressive alternative for sensitive patients. It is based on the manipulation of the needle by twisting, a classic practice in traditional Chinese medicine. Efficacy is evaluated through REL or referred pain, which indicates the correct localization of the PGM. If relief is not achieved, the direction of the needle can be changed and the procedure repeated (89, 90, 91, 92, 93).

For the mini-scalpel needle deep dry needling technique is compared to conventional acupuncture needles and self-stretching exercises, this technique has shown significantly superior results in the treatment of PGM. The thicker miniscalpel needle with a sharp tip is used in cases that do not respond to other treatments. However, more evidence is needed to justify its widespread use due to its more aggressive nature (89, 90, 91, 92, 93).

With respect to dry electropuncture, it acts through several mechanisms that justify its efficacy. Firstly, it is postulated that the electric current has the capacity to cause myocyte destruction around the needle, in addition to the mechanical injury already caused by the needle itself. However, it is important to note that this theory still needs to be validated by further research to determine the extent of this destruction and the dose required for it to occur. Another interesting mechanism is the washout of sensitizing substances. During the application of dry electropuncture, small but visible muscle contractions are achieved by slightly exceeding the excitomotor threshold. These contractions can facilitate a "washing out" effect on the sensitizing substances accumulated in the area, similar to what is observed in the relaxation techniques (REL) used in dry needling. In addition, the contractions provoked by the electric current also contribute to local stretching of the shortened sarcomeres at myofascial trigger points (MTrPs). This stretching helps to normalize muscle length, which in turn improves muscle function. Taken together, these mechanisms make dry electropuncture a promising tool in the treatment of muscle dysfunction (89, 90, 91, 92, 93).

4.2 Mechanisms and effects of PS.

4.2.1 Mechanisms of action of PS.

Superficial dry needling (SDP) and deep dry needling (DDP) are two techniques used in the treatment of myofascial pain, and although both involve the insertion of a needle, their mechanisms of action are different. PSS focuses on tissue surface stimulation without reaching myofascial trigger points (MTrPs), which leads to its effects not being justified solely by mechanical factors. Instead, it seeks to understand its efficacy through neurophysiology and endogenous mechanisms that modulate pain (56).

One of the most relevant mechanisms in PSS is the stimulation of A-beta nerve fibers, which are activated when the needle is inserted into the tissues above the PGM. This can block the transmission of nociceptive impulses coming from type IV muscle fibers, responsible for myofascial pain. This action can be direct, via inhibitory interneurons in the spinal cord, or indirect, via descending systems that use opioids, serotonin and noradrenaline to inhibit pain perception. In addition, diffuse inhibitory control of nociception is activated, which can also be activated by peripheral C-fibers, contributing to pain reduction (56).

The gate control theory, proposed by Melzack and Wall, suggests that stimulation of large-diameter A-beta nerve fibers closes the "gate" to pain transmission to the central nervous system. Although it has been revised over time, the essence of this theory persists and is considered fundamental to understanding how PSS can reduce pain perception. On the other hand, action on the autonomic nervous system is another mechanism under investigation. It has been found that this system can modulate the activity of PGMs, and animal studies suggest that sympathetic stimulation can increase the release of acetylcholine, which could contribute to decreased tension and improve the mobility of affected muscles (93).

With respect to PSP, this technique not only induces PSS, but also targets PGMs, eliciting responses that translate into additional mechanisms of action. One of the proposed mechanisms is the "washout" of sensitizing substances in the PGMs. By eliciting an endorphin release response (REL) via puncture, it has been shown to decrease the concentrations of compounds such as bradykinin and substance P, which are responsible for sensitization and perpetuation of pain. This "washout" may be related to an increase in blood flow that facilitates the elimination of these substances and improves motor plate physiology. Another mechanism of PSP is the elevation of pH in the PGM area, which is crucial, as an acidic pH is associated with pain sensitization. Studies show that after REL provocation, the pH of active PGMs rises, approaching normal muscle levels, which could help normalize motor plate function (56, 93, 94).

In addition, it has been proposed that stimulation of the PGM may interrupt the "PGM circuit", restoring the control that the central nervous system exerts over the affected area and contributing to the release of endorphins. It has also been observed that puncture can cause mechanical laceration of myocytes and motor plates, which may lead to regeneration and functional reorganization of the affected tissues (56, 93, 94).

Local stretching of contracted cytoskeletal structures is another mechanism that has been suggested, where the needle causes a stretch that may contribute to the normalization of sarcomere length, improving muscle function. Finally, the effects on blood flow and anti-inflammatory action following puncture are additional mechanisms that highlight the complexity of PSP. It has been observed that this technique can improve oxygenation and blood flow in muscles, which is essential to counteract the hypoxia that characterizes PGMs (56, 93, 94).

In summary, PSS and PSP present a number of mechanisms of action that go beyond the merely mechanical, involving complex interactions between the nervous, vascular and immune systems, which explains their analgesic and therapeutic effects in the treatment of myofascial pain. These findings invite further research on the efficacy and underlying mechanisms of these techniques, especially in terms of their comparison with placebo and their possible combination with other treatment modalities.

4.2.2 Effects on connective tissue.

In dry needling, thin, filiform needles are used to interact with the connective tissue of the body. The efficacy of these techniques is related to the small diameter of the needles (generally less than 300 mm), which allows for a specific interaction with the tissue, creating what is known as a "ball or swirl" of collagen around the needle. This phenomenon occurs when the needles are rotated, causing the collagen bundles to adhere and rotate with them, which increases the mechanical bond between the needle and the tissue. The mechanism of action is realized by (53, 93, 94, 95, 96):

- Needle rotation: By rotating the needle, a specific stretching of the connective tissue is generated, mainly affecting the subcutaneous and intermuscular layers, with minimal impact on the skin.
- Sustained stretch: When the needle is left in place after rotation, the collagen ball does not immediately unravel, allowing localized stretching to be maintained for several minutes.
- Measurement and quantification: Techniques, such as robotic acupuncture puncture and ultrasound elastography, have been developed to quantify connective tissue tangles and tissue displacements induced by needle manipulation.

Connective tissue constantly responds to mechanical forces, and this type of stimulation can induce viscoelastic responses depending on its composition and organization. Sustained stretching of the tissue beyond its usual range can lead to (53, 93, 94, 95, 96):

- Viscoelastic relaxation: Initially the tension in the tissue is reduced, followed by a molecular reorganization in the collagen matrix that restores the tension balance.
- Alterations in fibroblasts: These changes in cell shape (flattening and expansion) are active responses that may result in remodeling of the cytoskeleton and further reduction of tissue tension.

Although there is abundant evidence to suggest that manual needle stimulation influences the nervous system, there is still little knowledge about the mechanical link between the needle and the nervous system. The possibility that collagen coiling is an important mechanism for the transmission of mechanical signals is supported by studies where needle manipulation loses analgesic efficacy when the collagen-tissue link is disrupted. Some studies suggest a correspondence between acupuncture meridians and connective tissue, indicating that acupuncture points may be located in areas of denser or deeper connective tissue, which could explain differences in resistance to needle withdrawal at these points compared to control points (53, 93, 94, 95, 96).

4.2.3 Effects on muscle fascia.

The term "myofascial" was coined by Janet Travell in relation to trigger points (TP), which are hypersensitive areas in muscles that can generate referred pain. However, the scientific literature and Travell and Simons' seminal texts on PGs have tended to present muscles as isolated, self-contained structures with clearly defined origins and functions. This simplistic view does not reflect the complexity of the interrelationship between muscles and the fascial structures that surround them, a relationship that is crucial to understanding the etiology of myofascial pain. Fascia is classified into two main types: superficial fascia and deep fascia. Superficial fascia is composed of lax connective tissue, which lies just beneath the skin and contains collagen, elastin and adipose tissue. In contrast, the deep fascia is denser and surrounds muscles, nerves, blood vessels and organs, lacking adipose tissue. The separation between the deep fascia and the muscles is accomplished through a layer of lax connective tissue containing hyaluronan, a compound that facilitates sliding between the layers, essential to allow proper movement and reduce friction during muscle contraction (53, 93, 94, 95, 96).

The fascial layers surrounding the muscle are composed of epimysium, perimysium and endomysium. The epimysium envelops specific muscles and connects directly to the perimysium, which bundles bundles of muscle fibers. In turn, the endomysium wraps each muscle fiber individually, playing a vital role in flexibility and force transmission along the myofibrils. Tension in the deep fascia is maintained by numerous muscle insertions, allowing the muscles to distribute some of their contractile forces to the fascial structures. This interaction not only increases joint stability, but also facilitates coordinated movement between different muscle groups (53, 93, 94, 95, 96).

An interesting finding is that, although some muscles may have strong mechanical connections with their agonist muscles, force transmission is not always influenced by changes in the length of these muscles. This suggests that the mechanisms used to transmit force may vary between different muscles, further complicating our understanding of muscle and fascial function. In the context of dry needling, which involves inserting a needle into a PG, it is critical to consider how this procedure affects not only the PGs, but also the surrounding fascial structures. Dry needling resembles an injection treatment, and since the needle must pass through superficial and deep fascia to reach the PG, it is essential to investigate how these treatments interact with fascial structures. Langevin and colleagues have proposed that the rotation of solid filament needles may cause internal stretching in the tissues. They also suggested that there may be coupling between the needle and body tissues, possibly mediated by surface tensions and electrical attraction, although the latter may be relatively weak (96).

Myofascial pain is associated with the presence of tight bands, which are palpable perpendicular to the direction of the muscle fibers. This raises the hypothesis that restrictions in the fascia, particularly in the perimysium, could contribute to the formation of these tight bands. Indeed, the perimysium has been observed to respond to changes in mechanical tension more than other intramuscular connective tissues, indicating a significant relationship between fascia and the experience of pain. Recent research has suggested that modifications in lax connective tissue density in deep fascia, as well as hyaluronan hydrodynamics, may be contributing factors to the development of myofascial pain (53, 93, 94, 95, 96).

Despite the importance of the topic, research on the role of fascia in PGs and myofascial pain has been sparse. Many questions remain unanswered, such as what are the effects of dry needling on fascial adhesions, areas of densification, scar tissue, and the development of strength and flexibility. There is an urgent need for studies that define in detail the interactions between PGs, muscles and fasciae to better understand their role in myofascial pain. Understanding the relationship between fascia and trigger points is critical to developing more effective treatments. The interconnection between muscles and fascia is complex and must be integrated into clinical practice to adequately address pain associated with PGs. By recognizing the crucial role of fascial structures, healthcare professionals can optimize their therapeutic approach, potentially improving outcomes for their patients (53, 93, 94, 95, 96).

4.3 Principles and application procedures for correct practice in PS.

4.3.1 Medical history.

The medical history is the first essential step in ensuring effective treatment. In this process, the physical therapist must perform a thorough collection of patient information. This includes the medical history, documenting pre-existing conditions, past surgical interventions and any previous physiotherapeutic treatment received. In addition, it is essential to record current symptoms, detailing their nature, duration and location. A thorough physical assessment should also be carried out, analyzing range of motion, muscle strength and identification of trigger points. This information will allow the physiotherapist to decide the best therapeutic intervention to follow (97, 98).

4.3.2 Patient information and consent.

Once the clinical history has been collected, it is crucial to inform the patient about the proposed treatment. This information process should include a clear explanation of the dry needling technique: how it is performed and what the intended goals are. In addition, the physiotherapist should list the advantages of the treatment, such as pain reduction and improved mobility. However, it is also important to discuss the drawbacks and associated risks, such as post-procedural pain or possible bruising. By ensuring that the patient is well informed, a relationship of trust is created that will facilitate the process. Given the invasive nature of dry needling, it is essential to obtain the patient's consent. This consent must be informed, which means that the patient must fully understand what the procedure entails. It is recommended that, after explanation of the technique and its possible effects, the patient sign a consent document. This document not only ensures that the patient has understood the procedure, but also protects both the patient and the physical therapist in case of any eventuality (99, 100).

We must make a statement that I have received clear and understandable verbal information about the procedure to be performed on me and, furthermore, that I have read this document. All my doubts have been answered and I understand all the information provided. Therefore, I voluntarily give my consent for the physiotherapist specialized in dry needling to perform this technique on me. I also understand that I may withdraw my consent at any time without explanation. I will be offered a copy of this document upon request (101, 102).

Statement of informed consent for PS.	
PHYSIOTHERAPIST	
Name	
Surname	
Member no.	
Signature	
PATIENT	
Name	
Surname	
DNI	
Name and surname of the legal guardian (if applicable)	
Legal guardian's ID	
Signature	

Table 4. Model declaration of informed consent for SP (101, 102).

4.3.3 Hygiene.

Hygiene is a critical aspect in physical therapy practice, especially in invasive procedures. Prior to initiating the puncture, the physical therapist must comply with all established hygienic standards. This includes careful hand washing and, in many cases, the use of disposable gloves to create a barrier against any possible contamination. The patient's skin should also be disinfected in the area to be treated, using an appropriate antiseptic. Proper application of these rules ensures patient safety and reduces the risk of infection (103, 104).

4.3.4 Patient positioning.

Correct positioning of the patient is another vital aspect of a safe procedure. The physical therapist should ensure that the patient is in a comfortable prone position that allows easy access to the area to be treated. This position not only benefits the patient's comfort, but also allows the physical therapist to work more easily and safely. In addition, the use of cushions or supports can help ensure that the patient is as comfortable as possible during treatment (105, 106).

4.3.5 Diagnosis, localization and safe fixation of the PGM.

Before proceeding with the puncture, it is imperative to confirm the diagnosis and location of the muscle trigger point (MTrP). Without this step, the puncture could become an arbitrary procedure with unpredictable results. The physical therapist must ensure that the MTrP is correctly identified and fixed in a position that allows access during the puncture. This step is crucial, as it ensures that the treatment is specific and effective (107, 108).

4.3.6 Execution.

When the time comes to perform the puncture, it should be done with the greatest possible skill. Needle insertion should be done in a controlled manner, avoiding unnecessary depths to minimize risks. Throughout the process, it is essential to maintain constant communication with the patient, asking about their comfort and any symptoms they may be experiencing. This not only ensures that the patient feels safe, but also allows the physical therapist to adjust his or her technique as needed (107, 108).

4.3.7 Post-PS care.

Finally, once the puncture has been performed, certain care must be taken to ensure the patient's well-being. It is essential to apply hemostasis techniques to stop any bleeding at the puncture site. In addition, clear instructions should be provided to the patient on how to care for the treated area and what activities to avoid after the procedure. Adequate follow-up is equally important; scheduling a subsequent appointment allows the efficacy of the treatment to be evaluated and any side effects that may have arisen to be addressed (107, 108, 109, 110).

In terms of procedures, dry needling requires a detailed and meticulous approach to ensure both patient safety and treatment effectiveness. One of the first aspects to consider is patient positioning, which must be in a reclined position to avoid complications such as fainting during treatment. In addition, it is essential that the patient be positioned in a way that facilitates both palpation and adequate access to the muscle or group of muscles to be treated. The patient's position may vary between supine, prone, lateral, or a combination of these positions, depending on the location of the trigger points. Patient comfort is crucial, so pillows or other devices can be used to support and ensure patient relaxation. It is very useful for the clinician to be able to observe the patient's face during the dry needling session, as this facilitates fluid communication and allows assessment of the patient's reaction to the procedures. However, if this is not possible, verbal communication becomes an indispensable tool to detect any discomfort or warning signs from the patient. Likewise, the clinician must make sure to adopt an ergonomic posture, which not only allows him/her to perform the treatment efficiently but also to protect him/her from possible injuries or strains when applying the puncture. This body positioning helps to reduce risks associated with the technique and facilitates control of the entire process. In situations where the patient is a child, or if accompanied by other people, such as parents or guardians, it is important that they also feel comfortable. It is not uncommon that some accompanying persons may feel uncomfortable or even faint when observing the dry needling procedure, so the clinician must be prepared to manage these cases appropriately (107, 108, 109, 110).

Once the patient is properly positioned, we proceed with palpation, which is an essential step for the accurate identification of trigger points. Careful palpation allows localization of areas of pain and muscle tension, and for this, the clinician must have an excellent knowledge of anatomy. This knowledge encompasses muscle insertions, anatomical bony landmarks, the direction of muscle fibers, muscle layers, neurovascular structures and internal organs that could be at risk, such as the pleura or lungs, depending on the area being treated. The physical therapist must locate the muscle or muscles to be treated through a combination of visual observation and meticulous palpation. It is essential to avoid vulnerable anatomical structures such as nerves, blood vessels and important organs. Palpation must be precise to correctly identify trigger points, placing the muscle under optimal tension to facilitate this task. In some cases, the patient may be asked to contract the muscles to help the physical therapist better identify the directions of the muscle fibers and differentiate the muscles from each other. In terms of palpation technique, either a flat palpation or a pincer palpation technique may be chosen, depending on what is most appropriate for the area being treated. Forceps palpation is preferable in many cases, as it increases the safety of the procedure. Once the trigger point and muscle have been identified, and before proceeding with the puncture, it is important to ensure that both the patient and the muscle are completely relaxed. If the clinician has doubts about the precise location of the needle or about the patient's anatomy, especially in cases where obesity or other conditions complicate palpation, the clinician should not proceed with dry needling. When in doubt, it is always best to stop to avoid complications (107, 108, 109, 110).

The dry needling technique itself involves a series of specific steps that must be followed precisely. High-quality, sterile, single-use monofilament needles should be used. These needles may or may not be used with a guide tube, depending on clinician preference and patient needs. Needles should always be stored according to the manufacturer's guidelines and should not be expired. Needle length and gauge vary according to the patient's body size, the muscle to be treated and the depth required for the puncture. Prior to needle insertion, it is essential to follow a strict hygiene protocol. The clinician should wear gloves, at least on the hand performing the palpation, although gloves on both hands may be preferred. The muscle should be re-identified before the puncture, and a flat or pincer palpation technique can be used to ensure accuracy. The needle is held by the handle only and is inserted through the skin using the guide tube, which is removed once the needle is in place. It is essential to avoid touching the needle during the process to prevent contamination (107, 108, 109, 110).

The physical therapist must be thoroughly familiar with the anatomical structures near the area being treated. Avoiding penetration of vulnerable structures, such as nerves and blood vessels, is crucial. In addition, involuntary movements of the patient can compromise the safety of the puncture, so the clinician must keep a hand on the patient's body to control the situation. Depending on the dry needling technique being applied, such as superficial needling or deep needling, the needle will be inserted to the appropriate depth to reach the trigger point. In the case of deep needling, the needle is inserted slowly and continuously in and out of the muscle, known as the dynamic needling technique, with the aim of inducing local twitch responses (107, 108, 109, 110).

It is important to immediately discontinue the procedure if the patient experiences shooting, burning or electrical pain, as this could indicate that the needle has reached a nerve or blood vessel. In some cases, a static puncture technique may be used, where the needle is left in place for a specific period of time and may be rotated to apply mechanical stress on the fascia. Throughout the procedure, the clinician should maintain constant communication with the patient, adjusting the intensity of the treatment to the tolerance of himself. In particular, during the first treatment, it is essential to reassure the patient and ensure that the technique is tolerable and safe (107, 108, 109, 110).

After completing the treatment, proceed with the post-treatment phase. Immediately after removing the needle, the treated muscle should be compressed to control any bleeding, using a piece of cotton or gauze. If blood remains on the skin, it should be adequately cleaned with alcohol, and the materials used should be disposed of safely. The physical therapist should educate the patient about post-treatment care, which may include gentle stretching exercises, the use of warm or cold compresses, and possible modifications to daily activities. Finally, used needles should be disposed of immediately in a sharps-safe container, and follow local regulations for medical waste disposal. Safety and ongoing communication are fundamental pillars for the success of dry needling and patient satisfaction (107, 108, 109, 110).

4.4 Injuries caused by PS.

Dry needling (DP) is a technique used to treat myofascial pain syndrome, and is based on the abnormally high release of acetylcholine, which generates localized muscle contractures. These contractures, located just below or within a few microns of the synaptic area, are known as "active sites" in functional studies and "contraction nodes" in histological analysis. The accumulation of these active sites forms a myofascial trigger point (MTrP), which can be detected by palpation. PS seeks to eliminate these MTrPs to relieve pain symptoms, but its application can also cause damage to muscle and nerve fibers. The needles used in PS have a diameter ranging from 0.16 mm to 0.45 mm, considerably larger than that of myocytes, which on average is 40 μm. Needle insertion causes focal injury to the myocytes, classified as a laceration. To date, no studies have been performed on the cellular evolution of lesions caused by PS in muscles with PGM, so that the available data come from experiments in healthy rodent muscles, specifically the levator atri longus muscle, subjected to multiple punctures (111, 112, 113).

Muscle injury caused by PS is characterized by localized mechanical damage, which begins with a phase of degeneration caused by the inflammatory response. This cleansing phase is responsible for eliminating cellular debris, which is subsequently replaced by muscle regeneration. These degeneration, regeneration and repair processes occur simultaneously, although they are described separately in the text. The rupture of the muscle fiber membrane allows water to enter the cell, which causes cellular products to be released into the extracellular medium. PS also affects the blood vessels, resulting in extravasation of blood into the injured area. Intracellular substances activate mast cells in muscle tissue, which release chemokines into the bloodstream, attracting inflammatory cells. Initially, neutrophils are the predominant cells, followed by monocytes that become macrophages, responsible for phagocytosis of cellular debris. This process is specific, as it affects only necrotic debris and preserves the basal lamina, which serves as a support for viable satellite cells in the formation of new myofibers (111, 112, 113).

The accumulation of water in the injured area causes inflammation of the cisterns of the sarcoplasmic system, which store calcium for muscle contraction. Overhydration of these cisternae causes their rupture, releasing calcium which activates localized contractions in the area of injury and also acts on calcium-dependent proteases (CANP), which degrade the contractile apparatus. Over time, muscle regeneration becomes more evident, limited to the injured area by the formation of a contraction band that acts as a "firewall". This band prevents the spread of damage along the myocyte, ensuring that the majority of the muscle fiber remains intact (111, 112, 113).

The process of muscle regeneration is based on the activation of satellite cells, which are muscle stem cells located under the basal lamina of myocytes. These cells are activated after injury, becoming myoblasts, which multiply and enrich their membrane with calcium channels. Subsequently, the myoblasts fuse to form myotubes, assembling the new contractile apparatus with the surviving ends of the injured myocyte. This process may take about 7 days in minor injuries such as those caused by PS, during which time the regenerated muscle fibers tend to be atrophic, being referred to as young or immature muscle fibers. As normal contractile activity resumes, these fibers acquire adequate trophism. As muscle regeneration proceeds, fibroblasts synthesize proteins and proteoglycans to restore the extracellular matrix, essential for connective tissue integrity. Fibroblasts, which are resident cells in the endomysium, are activated by both mechanical aggression and intracellular substances released. Initially, they produce type III collagen, followed by type I collagen, which is difficult to eliminate and is broken down only into small fragments. Muscle contraction facilitates this elimination, and from the seventh day post-puncture, the collagen is segmented, being phagocytosed by inflammatory cells. Over time, the excess collagen is eliminated, restoring pre-injury conditions (111, 112, 113).

PS can cause axonal injury, resulting in distal segment degeneration and loss of function due to activation of axonal calpains, which degrade neurofilaments. The inflammatory reaction, mediated by macrophages, facilitates phagocytosis of axonal debris. After phagocytosis of the distal segment, the reinnervation process begins, where intracellular factors and mitogens promote axonal growth to reconnect with the postsynaptic component. The rate of reinnervation is 1-3 mm/day, crucial to restore neuromuscular function. However, complications such as aberrant connections can occur, and success depends on the health of the microenvironment and management of inflammation (111, 112, 113).

Dry needling causes a clean lesion in the axon, which favors rapid reinnervation due to the proximity between the site of lesion and the myocyte. The speed of reinnervation is linked to axoplasmic transport and preservation of the glial pathway, which facilitates the advancement of the axonal growth cone. Patient age is also an important factor, as regeneration tends to be impaired in older individuals. Although PS usually avoids damage to the active site of the nerve, it can affect muscle fibers outside the synaptic area. Studies in the levator auris longus muscle of mice have shown that, after multiple punctures, the inflammatory response intensifies in the first 24 hours, with almost complete muscle regeneration within 7 days. Intramuscular nerve injuries lead to rapid denervation of the postsynaptic component, followed by reinnervation within 3 days. In general, repetitive punctures do not adversely affect muscle regeneration and reinnervation processes (111, 112, 113).

5. ELECTRO-STIMULATION ON MYOFASCIAL TRIGGER POINTS

Percutaneous electrostimulation of myofascial trigger points (EPS) or dry electrostimulation (EPS) as a simpler and more practical alternative for clinical use. EPS consists of the application of electrical currents through needles inserted into myofascial trigger points (MTPs) to treat myofascial pain syndrome (MPS). Several important points are highlighted here (114, 115, 116, 117):

- Terminological differences: Although terms such as PENS (percutaneous electrical nerve stimulation), PNT (percutaneous neuromodulation therapy) and electroacupuncture are used in electrical stimulation techniques, the term EPS is distinguished because the needles are placed directly on the trigger points or on the tense band of the muscle, while in other techniques related areas such as dermatomes or traditional acupuncture points are stimulated.
- Treatment parameters: There is no clear consensus on the specific parameters for applying EPS, including needle location, current type, frequency, pulse duration, intensity and duration of treatment. These factors vary depending on the patient and the clinical experience of the therapist.
- Limited scientific evidence: despite some studies on EPS, there is little research and clinical trials that conclusively establish its effectiveness or optimal parameters. Many studies do not have sufficient methodological rigor (such as control groups or placebo), which makes it difficult to extrapolate results obtained in animals to humans.
- Application and adaptability: EPS can be customized according to the patient's needs, but this should be done with caution, respecting the contraindications, which will be detailed in other sections of the text.

This dry electropuncture approach is presented as a modern and precise technique within the invasive physiotherapy treatment of myofascial pain, differentiating it from other broader electrical stimulation techniques.

5.1 Parameters for the application of percutaneous electrical stimulation (PEEP) or dry electropuncture (EPS).

The recommended parameters for the application of dry electro-puncture (EPS) in the treatment of myofascial trigger points (MTrPs) include several aspects that should be adjusted according to the patient's needs and the observed therapeutic response. They are detailed here (114, 115, 116, 117):

5.1.1 Needle placement:

- Bipolar technique:
  - Two converging needles on the PGM
  - One needle in the PGM and one needle in the taut band outside the PGM.
  - One needle on each side of the PGM passing through the taut band, without passing through the PGM.
- Monopolar technique: Placement of a needle in the PGM connected to the negative electrode and an adhesive positive electrode nearby.

5.1.2 Waveform.

- Symmetric biphasic: recommended because it is better tolerated by patients and avoids adverse polar effects on tissues.
- Asymmetric biphasic or monophasic: they tend to generate discomfort due to the accumulation of ions under the needles, but have not been shown to affect pain relief.

5.1.3 Frequency.

- Combined frequencies (e.g., 2 Hz with 15 Hz or 2 Hz with 100 Hz), alternating every 2.5 to 3 seconds.
- Low frequencies (2 Hz): stimulate μ and δ opioid receptors, increasing the synthesis of enkephalins and endorphins.
- High frequencies (100 Hz): activate κ opioid receptors and stimulate the release of dynorphins.

5.1.4 Pulse width.

- High frequencies: use pulse width between 80-100 µs.
- Low frequencies: use pulse width between 200-250 µs.
- It must be adjusted to ensure a motor response without causing pain.

5.1.5 Intensity.

High intensity is recommended, causing a tapping or throbbing sensation along with a tolerable muscle contraction, but without pain.

5.1.6 Treatment time

- Maximum duration of 30 minutes per session to optimize the analgesic effect and avoid the development of tolerance.
- Longer applications (more than 30 minutes) may reduce the duration of analgesia.

5.1.7 Frequency of treatment:

2-3 sessions per week are considered optimal, adjusting according to the patient's response.

Dry needling should be applied in a personalized manner, based on these parameters and adjusted according to the patient's comfort and progress.

5.2 Contraindications of EEPP or EPS.

In addition to the general contraindications for dry needling, the following should be considered for EPS (114, 115, 116, 117):

- Cardiac pacemaker or arrhythmias: It is contraindicated, as electrical stimulation may interfere with pacemaker function or aggravate unstable arrhythmias. However, some studies have shown that EPS in remote areas (such as knees or elbows) does not generate detectable electrical fields in the chest.
- Pregnancy: It is absolutely forbidden during the first three months due to the risk of affecting the nervous and muscular system of the fetus. After the fourth month, some authors consider its use under supervision, avoiding the pelvis, abdomen and lumbar region.

- Active tumor processes: EPS is contraindicated in these conditions, as it could accelerate metastasis.
- Acute infections: It should not be applied in cases of active local infections, tuberculosis or septicemia.
- Unconscious patients: This is an absolute contraindication, as these patients cannot communicate discomfort or discomfort.
- Epilepsy: Strong or high frequency stimulation should not be applied, especially to the head. Stimulation in remote areas could be considered, but with extreme caution.
- Arterial hypertension: Intense stimulation should be avoided, especially with high frequencies, as it may aggravate the condition.
- Carotid sinus: EPS should not be applied to areas near the carotid sinus due to the risk of a sudden drop in blood pressure.
- Alterations in sensitivity: It should not be applied in areas with hyposensitivity or anesthesia, since the patient will not be able to perceive the electric currents.
- Thrombosis or thrombophlebitis: Avoid EPS in areas with thrombosis or thrombophlebitis to prevent the risk of embolism.
- Recent radiotherapy: Avoid applying EPS to areas treated with radiotherapy for at least 6 months after therapy due to tissue weakness.
- Infected wounds or skin lesions: Do not apply to these areas to avoid the spread of infection.

Bleeding: Stimulation may aggravate bleeding due to muscle contractions.

- Osteosynthesis: Avoid stimulation in areas where there are metallic implants, as it may generate strange or uncomfortable sensations.
- Head in children under 12 years of age: It is contraindicated due to the risk of convulsions.

EPS is a technique that uses electrical currents through needles to treat myofascial trigger points. It is recommended to use symmetrical biphasic waves, alternating frequency, pulse width between 100-250 μs and high intensity, without causing pain. Sessions should be 2-3 times per week, with a maximum of 30 minutes. Before its application, the contraindications of PS should be taken into account, as well as the specific contraindications that EEPP or EPS may have.

6. TREATMENT OF HYPERTONIA, SPASTICITY AND ALTERATIONS OF CENTRAL ORIGIN BY PS

The dry needling (DOT) technique has gained interest in neurological rehabilitation, although with few studies. Since 2004, Spanish physiotherapists have reported benefits of PSP in hypertonia and spasticity, suggesting a relationship between myofascial trigger points (MTrPs) and these conditions.

The Dry Needling for Hypertonia and Spasticity (DNHS) technique aims to reduce hypertonia and spasticity in patients with CNS lesions. Hypertonia is defined as increased muscle tone, with peripheral and central components. PGMs can exacerbate hypertonia by influencing biomechanics and sensory processing in the CNS. DNHS has shown improvements in motor control and functionality, and it is proposed that deactivating PGMs may improve sensorimotor processing. In conclusion, dry needling is presented as an effective tool to treat hypertonia and spasticity, complementing other treatments such as botulinum toxin. The DNHS technique was initially designed to address hypertonia and spasticity. However, its application has now been extended to look for more significant functional changes, relying on movement analysis and diagnostic tests such as electroencephalography (118, 119, 120, 121, 122).

As for the essential diagnostic criteria, these have been adapted from the identification of Myofascial Trigger Points (MTrPs). First of all, it is crucial to identlfy the tight bands in the accessible muscles, focusing on locating the one showing the highest degree of tension. Next, the existence of nodular areas is evaluated, paying attention to which of them is most sensitive. In addition, an assessment of the patient's movement and function is performed, which gives a clearer picture of the patient's condition. Finally, restriction in range of motion is considered, assessing both increased resistance to passive movement and triggering of myotatic reflexes. Confirmatory observations complement these criteria. Visual or tactile identification of a global twitch response (REG) or release (REL) is sought when the needle is inserted into the nodal area. Neural release is defined as a decrease in abnormal contractile activity of the muscle, which usually occurs after the onset of an REG or REL. Electromyography is also used to detect spontaneous electrical activity in the sensitive nodule (118, 119, 120, 121, 122).

As for the application procedure, the technique is performed following a series of adapted steps. First, the muscle is placed in a submaximal stretch position, which facilitates palpation and neural release. Then, the needle is probed for neural release, which usually occurs immediately after an ERW or REL. It is important to hold the needle in place for a short time until neural release is felt. Finally, the needle is withdrawn to the subcutaneous plane and insertion is repeated if necessary. The application guideline suggests maintaining an interval of 7 to 10 days between sessions to allow adequate repair of the neuromuscular lesions. Generally, improvements are evident during the first 3 to 4 treatment sessions, with more noticeable changes after the fifth or sixth session. Therefore, it is recommended to perform batches of 3 to 4 sessions, always ensuring a minimum of 7 days between each one. Subsequently, global reeducation work should be carried out to activate the musculature treated with the DNHS technique, thus allowing the beginning of a process of continuous improvement (118, 119, 120, 121, 122).

6.1 Indications and contraindications of DNHS.

DNHS is indicated for muscles with increased passive resistance, evaluated analytically, or for those that, after a functional assessment, hinder certain motor functions of the patient. This analysis considers myofascial trigger points (MTrPs) as activators or perpetuators of other MTrPs. Special attention is paid to the synergistic muscles of the affected muscle, acting as agonists or antagonists in a specific movement. The presence of PGMs in the affected muscle may result in overload or excitation/inhibition of related muscles, similar to what is seen in myofascial pain syndrome. In addition, the relationship between muscles sharing the same innervation or spinal segments is examined. According to the hypothesis of the DNHS technique, this may generate a neuromodulatory effect. The technique is applied to functionally altered muscles, their agonists and antagonists, as well as those sharing innervation, looking for a neuromodulatory effect. Conceptually, DNHS does not distinguish between active and latent PGMs, since pain is neither the main reason for consultation nor the objective of treatment. An order or hierarchy is established in the patient's evaluation, addressing muscles according to their importance within the constraints of time or pain caused by the puncture. However, since many patients tend to have several muscles affected, priority is given to treating those with increased resistance to passive movement, although there are studies that indicate the effectiveness of treating muscles without this characteristic, since they may be factors that activate or perpetuate others. As for the muscles that respond best to DNHS, they are those with abnormal muscle activity and exacerbated myotatic reflexes. Conversely, those whose evaluation suggests that resistance to passive stretch is due to soft tissue consolidation have a less favorable prognosis, as this situation is not indicative for DNHS (118, 119, 120, 121, 122).

Regarding resistance to passive movement, the effects are usually more significant and lasting in the upper limbs than in the lower limbs, possibly due to the load factor on the lower extremities. However, the greatest functional improvements are achieved in the lower limbs, especially in patients with better active mobility and functionality. It is considered easier to achieve functional improvements in the lower extremities due to their greater cerebral representation, especially in the hand (118, 119, 120, 121, 122).

Contraindications and risks of DNHS are similar to those of PGM puncture. For neurological patients, relative contraindications should be considered, such as sensory disturbances, use of anticoagulants and epilepsy. In such cases, a less aggressive initial treatment may be chosen to observe the patient's response. In certain situations, consultation with the patient's specialist physician is recommended to discuss the relevance of the contraindication (118, 119, 120, 121, 122).

6.2 Hypothesis and fundamentals of the DNHS technique.

We found 3 hypotheses based on the DNHS technique (118, 119, 120, 121, 122):

6.2.1 Hypothesis 1: Reprogramming and modification of afferent information.

Recent research suggests that, in cases of spasticity, the processing of afferent information at the spinal cord level is inadequate, which could be due to a decrease in presynaptic inhibition or to alterations in motor neuron inhibition. The idea that there is a problem in the information sent by the neuromuscular spindle has been ruled out and recurrent inhibition has been found to be normal in these patients. The DNHS® technique could facilitate the reprogramming of this information from skeletal muscle, which would improve processing and motor response.

6.2.2 Hypothesis 2: Neuromodulation of the central nervous system.

It is known that a sensitized system can present alterations such as a lower activation threshold to external stimuli. Dry needling could exert a neuromodulatory effect on sensitized systems, such as in patients with central nervous system (CNS) lesions. This could facilitate the opening of compensatory pathways, improving function. In addition, the technique could influence the myotatic reflex, which is directly related to spasticity and hypertonia, affecting both the muscle where the puncture is performed and other segmentally connected muscles.

6.2.3 Hypothesis 3: Active loci and muscle adaptations.

The presence of active loci in PGMs may be caused by an increase in acetylcholine (ACh), either by excess release or decreased acetylcholinesterase activity. In patients with upper motor neuron injury, this phenomenon may be related to hypersensitivity to denervation, which contributes to spasticity. This process is characterized by an increase of ACh receptors in the muscle fiber, increasing sensitivity to this neurotransmitter. The combination of increased ACh concentration and increased fiber sensitivity could explain the resistance to passive movement observed in these patients. The technique could ameliorate these factors by mechanically destroying myocytes and dysfunctional motor plaques, which would decrease ACh levels.

The dry needling technique for hypertonia and spasticity was developed from the application of dry needling on PGMs in patients with CNS lesions, with the aim of reducing hypertonia and spasticity. Although initially focused on the relationship between PGMs and these phenomena, its main focus is nowadays on improving the patient's functionality. Specific knowledge on indications, contraindications, diagnostic criteria and mechanisms of action has been established.

7. SPINAL CORD SEGMENTAL SENSITIZATION IN NEUROMUSCULOSKELETAL PAIN

Chronic pain syndromes, such as myofascial pain syndrome and fibromyalgia, involve neuroplastic changes that affect neuronal excitability and pain matrix structure, altering pain threshold and intensity. Activation of polymodal nociceptors may result in the release of neurotransmitters that facilitate central sensitization, affecting the balance between facilitatory and inhibitory mechanisms of pain. Myofascial trigger points are common causes of chronic neuromusculoskeletal pain (123, 124).

Segmental spinal sensitization (SES) is caused by hyperactivity of the dorsal horn following nociceptive impulses from damaged tissues. This manifests as allodynia and hyperalgesia in specific areas of the body. SES can persist regardless of the initial cause of pain, highlighting the importance of understanding segmental innervation for diagnosis and treatment. Myofascial pain arises from trigger points in tight muscles and is associated with peripheral and central sensitization. Although several substances are known to contribute to pain, the pathogenesis of myofascial pain is complex. Unlike acute pain, muscle pain is continuous, difficult to localize, and tends to cause neuroplasmic changes that can lead to chronicity (123, 124).

Sensitization, both peripheral and central, is responsible for the transition from normal to abnormal pain perception, which may persist without a noxious stimulus. Animal studies show that nociceptive afferents from skeletal muscle induce more significant neuroplastic changes in the spinal cord than those from cutaneous nociceptors. Continuous stimulation of muscle nociceptors can sensitize dorsal horn neurons, resulting in allodynia, hyperalgesia and referred pain. Sustained activation of nociceptors releases neurotransmitters such as L-glutamate and substance P, facilitating activation of previously inactive receptors. This causes central hyperexcitability, altering neuronal connectivity and expanding pain receptive fields in the spinal cord, with changes that can occur rapidly (123, 124).

Active PGMs present a specific biochemical milieu different from latent PGMs and healthy muscle. One study showed that patients with active PGMs in the upper trapezius had elevated levels of several endogenous pain-associated substances, such as substance P and CGRP, even in distant muscles. Furthermore, eliciting a local spasm response normalizes the concentration of these substances, suggesting that biochemical activity in PGMs may influence sensitization and persistent pain (123, 124).

Spinal facilitation refers to increased activity of neurons in the spinal cord due to the persistence of nociceptive stimuli in the dorsal horn. Normally, activation of primary nociceptors is regulated by inhibitory mechanisms, but continued activation can lead to the death of inhibitory neurons and sensitization of second-order neurons. This phenomenon is characterized by (125, 126):

- Increased flow in the ventral horn: Increases the activity of motor cells, raising muscle tone.
- Increased flow in the lateral horn: Generates autonomic reflexes that increase nociceptive activity.
- Increased flow in the dorsal horn: Produces electrical activity in the sensory nerve, known as "dorsal root reflexes".

These reflexes increase the production and release of neuropeptides such as substance P and CGRP, which can aggravate local inflammation, causing pain and hyperalgesia. In addition, adjacent spinal segments may become sensitized due to constant bombardment from the central nervous system. Noxious stimulation can destroy inhibitory neurons in one segment, which causes the nociceptive signal to activate neurons in this segment in future lesions, producing a recurrent pain pattern. This may lead to the sensation of "phantom pain" in excised organs, indicating that pain may persist due to changes in neuronal connectivity (125, 126).

Segmental Spinal Sensitization (SES) is commonly associated with musculoskeletal pain, playing a crucial role in the perpetuation of pain. For example, involvement of the thoracic levels (T1-T12) can facilitate and maintain abdominal pain and somatovisceral symptoms, which often mimic gastrointestinal diseases such as peptic ulcers. The development or activation of myofascial trigger points (MTrPs) is a manifestation of SES. Activation of these MTrPs may be temporary, often leading to recurrence of pain if segmental dysfunction is not addressed. SES is characterized by the presence of allodynia, hyperalgesia, and pressure sensitivity in specific areas innervated by a particular spinal segment (dermatome, myotome, and sclerotome). The diagnosis of SES involves (125, 126):

- Pain identification: The patient is asked to locate his or her pain and to evaluate its intensity on a scale of 1 to 10.
- Dermatome assessment: Techniques such as skin scraping are used to identify hyperalgesia or allodynia. The application of a pressure algometer helps to measure the Pressure Pain Threshold (PPU) in different muscles and areas.
- Myotome and sclerotome scan: Muscles and related structures are examined for PGMs and pain sensitivity.

Objective, quantifiable findings can guide the clinician in identifying the tissues involved in chronic pain and in understanding the severity of sensitization.

Treatment of SES involves identifying and desensitizing the affected spinal segment. This may include (125, 126):

- PS techniques: To treat primary or secondary sensitization.
- Identification of peripheral foci of nociception: The clinician should address and eliminate active PGMs and other generators of peripheral nociception that contribute to central sensitization.
- Ongoing evaluation: It is important to evaluate the effectiveness of treatment through subjective reduction of pain and objective improvements in segmental findings.

Effective management of SES in the clinic requires a comprehensive approach that combines identification of sensitized spinal segments and treatment of peripheral pain generators. This not only helps to relieve pain, but also improves the patient's function and quality of life (127, 128).

The paravertebral dry needling technique, developed by Fischer et al. focuses on the infiltration of 1% lidocaine into the paravertebral muscles, specifically between the spinous processes. This technique involves the use of a 0.45-mm diameter needle designed to reach the deep layers of the muscle without touching the vertebral lamina. Infiltration process (127, 128):

- Needle insertion: The needle is introduced in a sagittal direction through the paravertebral muscles, reaching maximum depth without touching the lamina.
- Aspiration: Before injecting, aspiration is performed to avoid blood vessels.
- Injection of anesthetic: Approximately 0.1 ml of lidocaine is injected and the needle is withdrawn and redirected caudally until reaching 5 mm of the reservoir.
- Repetition: This process is repeated in the cranial direction.

The benefits of PS:

- Less invasive: Acupuncture needles are less invasive than hypodermic needles, causing less inflammation and pain.
- Treatment of multiple segments: More segments can be treated at the same time, as they are not limited by the dose of local anesthetic.
- Increased Accuracy: Acupuncture needles provide better kinesthetic feedback, which facilitates manipulation and placement.

Although the technique shows positive results in pain reduction, scientific evidence remains limited. There are no double-blind, placebo-controlled clinical trials validating the effectiveness of paravertebral dry needling. However, studies have been proposed suggesting that dry needling may result in less postoperative pain and reduced analgesic requirements in patients undergoing arthroplasty (127, 128).

Paravertebral dry needling is a promising technique that could alleviate neuromusculoskeletal pain, especially in conditions of central sensitization. Understanding SES (segmental spinal sensitization) is crucial, as it helps to identify innovative treatments and address pain perpetuating factors. Combining treatments, including dry needling, can significantly improve patients' quality of life (127, 128).

8. PS OF NON-MYOFASCIAL TRIGGER POINTS (NMTP)

Dry needling (DP) refers to the insertion of a needle through the skin without the introduction of drugs, in contrast to infiltration which does involve the use of drugs. This chapter focuses on the PS of non-myofascial trigger points (NMTPs), while myofascial trigger points (MTrPs) are discussed in other chapters of the book. A classification of the different PS techniques is presented, followed by a definition of MTrPs and the most common treatment techniques (129, 130).

Theoretically, any spot that is painful to the touch and is not a PGM is classified as a PGNM. This includes (129, 130):

- Insertional trigger points in tendon attachment areas.
- Sore spots in sheaths, bursae, fasciae, and ligaments.
- Areas of injury due to trauma.
- Stitches in subcutaneous tissues.

PGNMs can be triggered by local spasm responses due to stimulation of an active PGM. Hong defines PGNMs as a set of sensitization foci, with sensitized nociceptors due to central or peripheral sensitization. PS at these foci can produce analgesia by hyperstimulation and relieve pain, sometimes using acupuncture points that are not painful (131, 132).

Regarding treatment, traditional Chinese acupuncture is one of the first techniques applied to treat PGNM, since many acupuncture points are Ah-Shi points, which are located in non-muscular tissues. When applying acupuncture, the needle can be rotated or electrical stimulation can be applied to increase efficacy. Other techniques in the treatment of PGNM include (131, 132):

- PS with multiple rapid insertions: Originally used by Travell to infiltrate PGMs, this technique involves multiple rapid needle insertions to localize and desensitize nociceptors. It seeks to stimulate a greater number of sensitized nociceptors by rapid movement, avoiding tissue damage and causing immediate pain relief.

- PS for soft tissue release: This technique focuses on soft tissue manipulation to release tension and pain.
- PS with electrostimulation: Combines PS with electrical stimulation to enhance the analgesic effect.
- Superficial PS: Applies PS to the surface of the skin, similar to acupuncture, although it generally does not provide complete immediate pain relief.
- PGNM PS, especially through the multiple rapid insertion technique, focuses on relieving pain by treating the underlying source of pain, rather than focusing solely on the PGM.

8.1 Mechanisms of PS in PGNM.

Dry needling (DP) is a therapeutic technique that uses needles to treat trigger points, with the aim of relieving pain. Several mechanisms have been proposed to explain how SP can achieve this relief (131, 132):

- Downstream pain inhibitory system: This system is an intrinsic mechanism of the body that controls pain. It is suggested that both hyperstimulation analgesia and disruption of the "PGM circuit" act through this system. According to Melzack, hyperstimulation analgesia is the main therapeutic mechanism of acupuncture for pain relief. During PS, local spasm responses (REL) are generated, which are essential for immediate and complete pain relief (93).
- Interruption of the vicious circle: Hong proposes that the main mechanism of PS is to interrupt the vicious circle of the PGM circuit, which could also include the connection of PGNMs to trigger point circuits in the spinal cord.
- Stimulation of nociceptors: When PS is performed, nerve impulses are sent to the dorsal horn cells of the spinal cord, which can break the vicious circle of the PGM circuit. Vigorous stimulation of sensitive loci (sensitized nociceptors) is key to achieving optimal pain relief.

8.2 Application of the PS technique for PGNM.

The following practical considerations should be taken into account (133, 134):

- Type of needles: The use of hypodermic needles with the following sizes is recommended:
  - 0.50 mm x 40 mm for normal use.
  - 0.60 mm x 70 mm for thick or deep tissues.
  - 0.40 mm x 30 mm for thin and superficial tissues.
  - Acupuncture needles can also be used, although they are more difficult to handle and require practice. The needles must be thicker than 0.30 mm.
- Insertion Technique: Before performing the puncture, it is essential to ensure that other non-invasive therapies have been explored and that any pathological lesions responsible for the pain have been removed. During the puncture the needle is directed towards the most sensitive region, moving rapidly inwards and outwards. Any lateral movement should be avoided, ensuring that the needle tip contacts as many sensitized nociceptors as possible. The needle insertion speed should be approximately 20-30 mm/s.
- Post-procedure: After puncture, compression should be applied to the penetration site to avoid excessive bleeding and reduce post-puncture pain.

8.3 Types of PS techniques in PGNM.

Regarding the types of techniques we can find (133, 134):

- Rapid entry and exit technique with rotation: Chou et al. have developed a recent technique known as "rapid entry and exit with rotation" using acupuncture needles. Because acupuncture needles are flexible and their small gauge makes rapid movement difficult, Chou incorporated needle rotation (coiling) to facilitate the movement in and out, preventing bending during the procedure. This technique is especially useful in people with fibromyalgia, as the small diameter of the needle minimizes tissue irritation, reducing pain and post-puncture discomfort, which often lasts several days in these patients. For its procedure the technique is performed with acupuncture needles. Rapid entries and exits are performed with simultaneous rotation of the needle to avoid bending.

- PS for soft tissue release: To treat chronic musculoskeletal problems that do not respond to physical therapy or infiltrations, surgical intervention or minimally invasive techniques are often required. Among these techniques is dry needling for soft tissue release. Lin's technique has developed a less invasive technique to release adherent soft tissues by using a blunt cannula to simultaneously inject hyaluronic acid and local anesthetic. Alternatively, a normal dry needle puncture can be used if applied slowly. With regard to the procedure the needle penetrates the skin and advances slowly into the painful region. In addition, a lateral movement is performed to release soft tissue adhesions. The presence of pain or resistance to the movement of the needle indicates the location of the adhesions. Once the resistance decreases, the needle is withdrawn into the subcutaneous layer and redirected to penetrate in different trajectories to release the adherent tissues extensively. This technique is effective for releasing tendon adhesions, often related to insertional myofascial trigger points (MTrPs). The most common adhesions that can be treated include the rotator cuff tendons, the biceps brachii tendons, the forearm extensor and flexor muscles at the elbow, and the quadriceps tendon and patellar ligament.

Dry needling techniques with rapid entry and exit with rotation, and dry needling for soft tissue release, are effective approaches to treat non-myofascial trigger points (NMTPs). These techniques can trigger hyperstimulation analgesia and, when performed properly, can relieve pain and release adhesions in tissues such as tendons, ligaments and fascia.

BIBLIOGRAPHIC REFERENCES

1. Simons, D.G., Travell, J.G., Simons, L.S. (2002). Myofascial pain and dysfunction: The trigger point manual. Upper half of the body, 2ed. Madrid: Editorial Médica Panamericana. ISBN: 9788479035754.
2. Simons D.G. (2004). New aspects of myofascial trigger points: etiological and clinical. J Musculoskelet Pain. 12(3-4): 15-21.
3. Iturriga, V., Bornhardt, T., Hermosilla, L. and Avila, M. (2014). Prevalence of Myofascial Pain in Masticatory and Cervical Muscles in a Center Specializing in Temporomandibular Disorders and Orofacial Pain. Int. J. Odontostomat, 8(3), 413-417.
4. Muñoz, J.P., Alpizar, E. (2016). Myofascial syndrome. Medicina legal de Costa Rica. 33(1).
5. Fleckenstein, J., Zaps, D., Ruger, L.J., Lehmeyer, L., Freiberg, F., Lang, P.M., etal. (2010). Discrepancy between prevalence and perceived effectiveness of treatment methods in myofascial pain syndrome: results of a cross-sectional, nationwide survey. BMC Musculoskelet Disord. 11: 11-32.
6. Chien, J.J., Bajwa, Z.H. (2008). What is mechanical back pain and how best to treat it? Current Pain and Headache Reports, 12(5): 406-411.
7. Fernández, C., Alonso, C., Miangolarra, J.C. (2007). Myofascial trigger points in subjects presenting with mechanical neck pain: A blinded, controlled study. Manual Therapy. 12(1): 29-33.
8. Sanita, P., De Alentar, F. (2009). Myofascial pain syndrome as a contributing factor in patients with chronic headaches. Journal of Musculoskeletal Pain. 17(1): 15-25.
9. Borg-Stein, J. (2002). Cervical myofascial pain and headache. Current Pain and Headache Reports. 6(4): 324-330.
10. Lucas, K., Rich, P., Polus, B. (2008). How common are latent myofascial trigger points in the scapular positioning muscles? Journal of Musculoskeletal Pain. 16(4): 279-286.

11. Affaitati, G., Costantini, R., Fabrizio, A., et al. (2011). Effects of treatment of peripheral pain generators in fibromyalgia patients. European Journal of Pain, 15(1): 61-69.

12. Mayoral, O., Salvat, I. (2021). Invasive physiotherapy of myofascial pain syndrome. Editorial médica panamericana. ISBN: 978-8491103950.

13. Martínez, J.M., Pecos, D. (2005). Diagnostic criteria and clinical features of myofascial trigger points. Fisioterapia. 27(2): 65-68.

14. Ruiz, M., Nadador, V., Fernández, J., Hernández, J., Riquelme, I., Benito, G. (2007). Pain of muscular origin: myofascial pain and fibromyalgia. Revista sociedad española del dolor. 1: 36-44.

15. Estevez, E.A. (2001). Myofascial pain. MedUnab. 4(12).

16. Hernández, F.M. (2009). Myofascial syndromes. Clinical Rheumatology. 5(S2): 36-39.

17. Diaz, L. (2014). Myofascial cervicalgia. Clinical medical journal condes. 25(2): 200-208.

18. Niel, S. The concise book of trigger points: Professional and self-help manual (2017). Editorial Paidotribo. ISBN: 9788499106038

19. Hernández, F.M. (2009). Myofascial syndromes. Clinical Rheumatology. 5(S2): 36-39.

20. Simons, D.G. (1999). Diagnostic criteria of myofascial pain caused by trigger points. Journal of Musculoskeletal Pain. 7(1-2):111-20.

21. Hong, C.Z., Kuan, T.S., Chen, J.T., Chen, S.M. (1997). Referred pain elicited by palpation and by needling of myofascial trigger points: acomparison. Arch Phys Med Rehabil. 78(9):957-60.17.

22. Hong, C., Chen, Y.N., Twehous, D.A., Hong, D.H. (1996). Pressure threshold for referred pain by compression on the trigger point andadjacent areas. J Musculoske Pain. 4(3):61-79.

23. Moldofsky, H. (2001). Sleep and pain. Sleep Medicine Reviews. 5: 387-398.

24. Gil, E., Martínez, G.L., Aldaya, C., Rodriguez, M.J. (2007). Myofascial pain syndrome of the pelvic girdle. Revista sociedad española dolor. 5: 358-368.

25. González, I., Varas, A.B., García, S. (2003). Objective evaluation of muscle tissue after treatment of myofascial trigger points: A study of 20 cases. Revista iberoamericana fisioterapia kinesiología. 6(3): 109-123.

26. Araya, F., Rubio, D., Gutiérrez, H., Arias, L., Olguín, C. (2018). Dry needling and changes in muscle activity in subjects with myofascial trigger points: case series. Journal of the Spanish pain society.

27. Delaune, V. (2013). Trigger points: treatment for pain relief. Paidotribo. ISBN: 9788499109015

28. Borg, J., Simons, D. (2002). Myofascial Pain. Focused Review. 83(1): S40-47.

29. Tough, E.A., White, A., Richards, S., Campbell, J. (2007). Variability of criteria used to diagnose myofascial trigger point pain Syndrome-Evidence from a review of the literature. The Clinical Journal of Pain. 23(3): 278-286.

30. Wolfe, F., Clauw, D., Fitzcharles, M., Goldenberg, R., Katz, R., Mease. P., et al. (2010). The American College of Rheumatology preliminary diagnostic criteria for fibromyalgia and measurement of symptom severity. 62(5): 600-610.

31. Ruiz, M., Nadador, V., Fernández, J., Hernández, J., Riquelme, I., Benito, G. (2007). Pain of muscular origin: myofascial pain and fibromyalgia. Spanish Pain Society Journal. 1: 36-44

32. Dommerholt, J., Fernandez, C. (2018). Trigger Point Dry Needling: An Evidenced and Clinical-Based Approach. 2nd edition. Elselvier. ISBN: 978-0702074165.

33. Dommerholt, J., Bron, C., Franssen, J. (2011). Myofascial trigger points: an evidence-informed review. The Journal of Manual and Manipulative Therapy. 14(4): 203-221.

34. Dommerholt, J., Mayoral, O., Gröbli, C. (2006). Trigger Point Dry Needling. The Journal of Manual and Manipulative Therapy. 14(4): 70-87.

35. Shah, J.P., Gilliams, E.A. (2008). Uncovering the biochemical milieu of myofascial trigger points using in vivo microdialysis: An application of muscle pain concepts to myofascial pain syndrome. The journal of bodywork and movement therapies. 12(4): 371-384.

36. Sikdar, S., Shah, J.P., Gebreab, T., Yen, R.H., et al. (2009). Novel applications of ultrasound technology to visualize and characterize myofascial trigger points and surrounding soft tissue. Archives of Physical Medicine and Rehabilitation. 90: 829-838.

37. Niraj, G., Collet, B.J., Bone, M. (2011). Ultrasound-guided trigger point injection: first description of changes visible on ultrasound scanning in the muscle containing the trigger point. British journal of anesthesia. 107: 474-475.

38. Rha, D.W., Shin, J.C., Kim, Y.K., Jung, J.H., et al. (2011). Detecting local twitch responses of myofascial trigger points in the lowerback muscles using ultrasonography. Archives of Physical Medicine and Rehabilitation. 90: 1576-1580.

39. Lewis, J., Tehan, P.A. (1999). Blinded pilot study investigating the use of diagnostic ultrasound for detecting active myofascial trigger points. Pain. 79: 39-44.

40. Chen, Q., Bensamoun, S. F., Basford, J. R., Thompson, J. M., An, K. N., Ehman, R. L. (2007). Identification and quantification of myofascial taut bands with magnetic resonance elastography. Archives of Physical Medicine and Rehabilitation. 88(12): 1658-1661.

41. Feng, S., Zhang, Z., Xu, S., Han, P., Yang, J. (2018). Ultrasonic elastography in the evaluation of myofascial trigger points. BioMed Research International. 1-8.

42. Turo, D., Otto, P., Shah, J. P., Heimur, J., Sikdar, S. (2015). Ultrasonic characterization of the upper trapezius muscle in patients with myofascial pain syndrome using acoustic radiation force impulse imaging and shear wave elastography. Journal of Ultrasound in Medicine. 34(12): 2149-2160.

43. Sikdar, S., Shah, J. P., Gilliams, E. A., Gebreab, T., Gerber, L. H. (2009). Assessment of myofascial trigger points using ultrasound imaging and vibration sonoelastography. Archives of Physical Medicine and Rehabilitation. 90(11): 1829-1838.

44. Turo, D., Cassar, T., Harshbarger, D., Gebreab, T., Otto, P., Shah, J. P., et al. (2013). Ultrasonic characterization of the upper trapezius muscle in patients with chronic neck pain. Ultrasound in Medicine and Biology. 39(12): 2520-2530.

45. Zhou, K., Hong, Y., Huang, Z., Tang, C., Wang, H., Zhou, Q. (2014). Characterization of myofascial trigger points in patients with upper trapezius pain using ultrasound imaging. Journal of Rehabilitation Research and Development. 51(6): 901-910.

46. Shah, J.P., Gilliams, E.A. (2008). Uncovering the biochemical milieu of myofascial trigger points using in vivo microdialysis: An application of muscle pain concepts to myofascial pain syndrome. The Journal of Bodywork and Movement Therapies. 12(4): 371-384.

47. Chen, Q., Basford, J.R., An, K.N. (2011). Ability of magnetic resonance elastography to assess taut bands. Clinical Biomechanics. 26(6): 610-615.

48. Jiang, W., Huang, Z., Yang, H., Wang, H., Zhou, K. (2015). MRI and ultrasound imaging of myofascial trigger points. American Journal of Physical Medicine and Rehabilitation. 94(1): 34-40.

49. Reeves, J.L., Jaeger, B., Graff. S.B. (1986). Reliability of the pressure algometer as a measure of myofascial trigger point sensitivity. Pain, Elsevier. 24(3): 313-321.

50. Fischer, A.A. (1987). Letter to the editor. Pain, Elsevier. 28(3): 411-414.

51. Huang, Q.M., Ma, Y.T., Li, W. (2010). Assessment of myofascial trigger points using infrared thermography: A systematic review. Complementary Therapies in Medicine. 18(3-4): 144-149.

52. Sikdar, S., Shah, J.P., Gebreab, T. (2011). Quantitative assessment of myofascial trigger points from thermographic images using advanced image processing techniques. Journal of Bodywork and Movement Therapies. 15(2): 158-164.

53. Hidalgo, J., Torres, M., Mayoral, O., Sanchez, Z., Prieto, S. (2013). Infrared thermography for the detection of myofascial trigger points in patients with neck pain. Medical Physics. 40(7).

54. Alkhatib, B., Sultan, M.A. (2011). Infrared thermography in the detection of active myofascial trigger points. Journal of Medical Engineering and Technology. 35(6-7): 311-318.

55. American Physical Therapy Association (APTA). (2012). Physical therapists and the performance of dry needling. 1-141.

56. Baldry, P. (2005). Acupuncture, trigger points and musculoskeletal pain. 3rd ed. Churchill Livingstone. ISBN: 978-0443066443.

57. Hong, C.Z. (1994). Lidocaine injection versus dry needling to myofascial trigger points: The importance of the local twitch response. American Journal of Physical Medicine and Rehabilitation. 73(4): 256-263.

58. Cummings, T.M., White, A.R. (2001). Needling therapies in the management of myofascial trigger point pain: A systematic review. Archives of Physical Medicine and Rehabilitation. 82(7): 986-992.

59. Tough, E.A., White, A.R., Cummings, T.M., Richards, S.H., Campbell, J.L. (2009). Acupuncture and dry needling in the management of myofascial trigger point pain: A systematic review and meta-analysis of randomized controlled trials. European Journal of Pain. 13(1): 3-10.

60. Kietrys, D.M., Palombaro, K.M., Azzaretto, E. (2013). Effectiveness of dry needling for upper-quarter myofascial pain: A systematic review and meta-analysis. Journal of Orthopaedic and Sports Physical Therapy, 43(9): 620-634.

61. Peuker, E.T., White, A. (1999). Anatomy for the clinical practice of acupuncture. Clinical Anatomy. 12(3): 174-182.

62. Ernst, E., White, A.R. (2001). Prospective studies of the safety of acupuncture: A systematic review. American Journal of Medicine. 110(6): 481-485.

63. Cummings, T.M., Baldry, P. (2007). Regional myofascial pain: Diagnosis and management. Best Practice and Research Clinical Rheumatology. 21(2): 367-387.

64. Aldlyami, E., Kulkarni, A., Reed, M.R., Muller, S.D. (2010). Partington Latex-free gloves: safer for whom? J. Arthroplasty. 25: 27-30.

65. Mayoral, O. (2009). Trigger point dry needling: A simple technique for the treatment of myofascial pain. Fisioterapia. 31(3): 126-134.

66. Ernst, E., White, A. (2001). Acupuncture and dry needling safety review: Infection risks and prevention. American Journal of Medicine. 110(6): 481-485.

67. Peuker, E.T., White, A. (1999). Anatomical considerations and needle safety in acupuncture. Clinical Anatomy. 12(3): 174-182.

68. Dann, J.J., Eckstein, M. (1992). The occurrence of infections with skin punctures: A prospective study of 5,000 punctures without skin preparation. Journal of Clinical Medicine. 8(4): 405-411.

69. Wit, M.J., Johnson, L.C., Baker, S.J. (1997). Risk of infections in trigger point dry needling: A review of 230,000 cases. Acupuncture in Medicine. 15(1): 35-40.

70. Zhang, X., Li, J., Zhou, Q. (2009). Infections in acupuncture and dry needling: Bacterial and viral complications. Chinese Journal of Traditional Medicine. 15(3): 21-28.

71. Rosenblatt, M.A., Abelson, S.A. (2005). Complications and safety considerations in acupuncture and dry needling: Puncture accidents and risk management. Pain Medicine. 6(1): 53-59.

72. García, M. J., López, R. A. (2022). Dry needling considerations: contraindications and precautions. Journal of Physical Therapy and Rehabilitation. 34(2): 123-130.

73. Fernandez, A. L., Torres, S. (2021). Effects of dry needling in patients with complex medical conditions. Journal of Pain Management. 29(4): 45-54.

74. Martinez, P. (2020). Manual therapy and dry needling: a practical guide for the physical therapist. Editorial Médica Panamericana.

75. Sanchez, T., Ruiz, J. (2019). Physical therapy and pain management: contemporary approaches. Elsevier.

76. Perez, L. (2020). Contraindications in dry needling therapy. Advances in physiotherapy. Springer. 245-260.

77. Morales, E. (2018). Assessment and risks in dry needling. In S. Fernandez (Ed.), Contemporary therapies in chronic pain. Editorial Médica. 115-130.

78. Rodriguez, A. (2021). Evaluation of the effectiveness and safety of dry needling in patients with muscle pain: a clinical study. Master's thesis, University of Barcelona.

79. Boyce, J.M., Pittet, D. (2002). Guideline for hand hygiene in health-care settings: Recommendations of the Healthcare Infection Control Practices Advisory Committee and the HICPAC/SHEA/APIC/IDSA Hand Hygiene Task Force. American Journal of Infection Control 30(8): S1-S46.

80. Health Service Executive (HSE). (2009). Standard precautions in health care. Health protection surveillance centre.

81. Strategy for the Control of Antimicrobial Resistance in Ireland (SARI). (2005). Guidelines for hand hygiene in Irish healthcare settings.

82. Ehrenkranz, N.J., Alfonso, B.C. (1991). Failure of bland soap handwash to prevent hand transfer of patient bacteria to urethral catheters. Infection Control and Hospital Epidemiology. 12(11): 654-662.

83.Paulson, D.S., Riccelli, E., Fendler, E. (1999). A comparison of the antimicrobial activity of plain soap, antimicrobial soap, and an alcoholic hand gel. Infection Control and Hospital Epidemiology. 20(6): 396-401.

84.Center for Disease Control and Prevention (CDC). (2019). Guideline for infection control in healthcare personnel. Morbidity and Mortality Weekly Report. 68(3): 1-32.

85.Health Service Executive (HSE). (2009). Use of personal protective equipment (PPE) in healthcare settings.

86.World Health Organization (WHO). (2019). Best practices for injections and related procedures toolkit. WHO Guidelines on Injection Safety.

87.World Health Organization (WHO) (2009). WHO guidelines on hand hygiene in health care: First global patient safety challenge clean care is safer care.

88.Yunus, M.B., and Mense, S. (2019). Myofascial pain syndrome and trigger points: clinical review and pathophysiology. Pain Medicine. 21(2): 179-190.

89.Cagnie, B., Dewitte, V., Barbe, T., Timmermans, F., Delrue, N. (2020). Needling therapies in the management of myofascial trigger points: A systematic review. American Journal of Physical Medicine and Rehabilitation. 99(4): 309-318.

90.Gattie, E., Cleland, J.A., Snodgrass, S.J. (2017). Dry needling for patients with musculoskeletal pain: A clinical commentary. International Journal of Sports Physical Therapy. 12(2): 227-236.

91.Kietrys, D. M., Palombaro, K. M., Azzaretto, E. (2019). Effectiveness of dry needling for upper-quarter myofascial pain: A systematic review and meta-analysis. Journal of Orthopaedic and Sports Physical Therapy. 43(9): 620-634.

92.Shah, J. P., Thaker, N. (2018). Myofascial pain and nociceptive trigger points: Time to integrate dry needling with evidence-based medicine. The Journal of Orthopaedic and Sports Physical Therapy. 48(1): 3-9.

93. Melzack, R., Wall, P.D. (1965). Pain mechanisms: a new theory. Science, 150(3699): 971-979.

94. Dommerholt, J., Fernández-de-las-Peñas, C. (2013). Trigger Point Dry Needling: An Evidence and Clinical-Based Approach. Churchill Livingstone.

95. Shah, J.P., Gilliams, E.A. (2008). Uncovering the biochemical milieu of myofascial trigger points using in vivo microdialysis: An application of muscle pain concepts to myofascial pain syndrome. Journal of Bodywork and Movement Therapies. 12(4): 371-384.

96. Langevin, H.M., Yandow, J.A. (2002). Relationship of acupuncture points and meridians to connective tissue planes. The Anatomical Record. 269(6): 257-265.

97. Dutton, M. (2018). Fundamentals of Musculoskeletal Assessment Techniques. 4th ed. New York: Elsevier.

98. Kettner, N., Ragnarsdottir, M. (2014). The Importance of Medical History and Physical Examination in the Clinical Setting. Journal of Physical Therapy Science. 26(4): 649-653.

99. Gillon, R. (2015). Informed Consent: A Guide for Healthcare Professionals. Journal of Medical Ethics. 41(5): 391-395.

100. Riazi, H., Dyer, C. B. (2016). Informed Consent: Ethical and Legal Considerations in Physical Therapy Practice. Physiotherapy Theory and Practice. 32(1): 37-46.

101. Groves, M. (2016). Documenting Informed Consent In Physical Therapy: An Ethical and Legal Imperative. Journal of Physical Therapy Education. 30(3): 15-22.

102. Schenck, K.L., Hall, R.M. (2018). Legal Considerations in Informed Consent for Physical Therapy. Journal of Legal Medicine. 39(3): 331-344.

103. McEwen, I.R., Pomeranz, B. (2015). Clinical Handbook of Physiotherapy. New York: Wiley.

104. Walker, J.A., Allen, S.S. (2017). Infection Control in Physical Therapy Practice. Journal of Physical Therapy Science. 29(9): 1665-1670.

105. Glover, J.E., Pomeranz, B. (2016). Patient Positioning and Ergonomics in Rehabilitation. Physical Therapy. 96(5): 617-626.

106. Sweeney, J., Murphy, A. (2019). Best Practices for Patient Positioning in Manual Therapy Techniques. Physiotherapy Theory and Practice. 35(2): 136-142.

107. Cummings, T.M., Cummings, T.J. (2015). Dry Needling: A Clinical Perspective. Journal of Manual and Manipulative Therapy. 23(3): 145-155.

108. Dommerholt, J. (2011). Myofascial Trigger Points: Pathophysiology and Evidence-Informed Diagnosis and Management. Journal of Manual and Manipulative Therapy. 19(3): 137-147.

109. Trevelyan, F.C., and Noyes, R.A. (2018). Post-Needling Care: Understanding the Role of Patient Education. Physical Therapy Reviews. 23(1): 22-31.

110. Dunning, J. et al. (2014). Dry Needling: A Comprehensive Review of the Literature. Acupuncture in Medicine. 32(3): 207-215.

111. Alvarez, A. (2015). Dry needling: efficacy in the treatment of myofascial pain syndrome. International Journal of Medicine and Sciences of Physical Activity and Sport. 15(59): 245-258.

112. Sato, T., Rosen, J. (2020). Effects of dry needling on muscle pain: a systematic review. Physiotherapy Theory and Practice. 36(4): 428-441.

113. Ursini, T., Tontodonati, M. (2018). The role of inflammation in muscle regeneration. Current Opinion in Rheumatology. 30(1): 38-43.

114. Bae, H., Kim, J. H., Lee, H. (2020). The effectiveness of dry needling for myofascial trigger points: A systematic review and meta-analysis. Archives of Physical Medicine and Rehabilitation. 101(9): 1626-1638.

115. López-de-Silva, M., et al. (2021). Electroacupuncture versus dry needling for myofascial pain syndrome: A randomized controlled trial. Pain Medicine. 22(1): 123-130.

116. Huang, Y., et al. (2023). Efficacy of dry needling combined with electrical stimulation for myofascial pain syndrome: A systematic review and meta-analysis. Pain Medicine. 24(2): 331-340.

117. Kumar, S., Dhanjal, M. (2023). Effects of electroacupuncture and dry needling on myofascial pain: A randomized controlled trial. Journal of Bodywork and Movement Therapies. 30: 234-240.

118. García, A., Peñas, C. (2023). Efficacy of dry needling in myofascial pain syndrome: A systematic review and meta-analysis. Journal of Rehabilitation Medicine. 55(1).

119. Klein, A.J., Cohen, M.L. (2021). Trigger point dry needling: A systematic review of the evidence. Archives of Physical Medicine and Rehabilitation. 102(10): 1852-1860.

120. López, I., et al. (2020). Effectiveness of dry needling for myofascial pain: A systematic review and meta-analysis. Physical Therapy Reviews. 25(4): 237-250.

121. Teodorczyk, J.A., Injeyan, H.S. (2021). Efficacy of dry needling in patients with chronic musculoskeletal pain: A narrative review. Pain Research and Management. 1-9.

122. González, M., Peñas, C. (2022). Dry needling in neuromuscular rehabilitation: A systematic review. Physiotherapy Theory and Practice. 38(2): 194-206.

123. Böning, R., Marziniak, M. (2020). Central sensitization in chronic pain: A review. Pain Physician. 23(1): 17-26.

124. Klein, A.J., Cohen, M.L. (2022). Dry needling for myofascial trigger points: A systematic review and meta-analysis. Archives of Physical Medicine and Rehabilitation. 103(3): 513-524.

125. Aukerman, M.A., et al. (2020). The role of neuroplasticity in chronic pain syndromes. Pain Management. 10(5): 325-332.

126. Marquez, R.L., Rios, J. (2021). The effects of dry needling on myofascial pain syndrome: A review of the literature. NeuroRehabilitation. 49(1): 1-11.

127. Jiang, Y., et al. (2023). Effects of dry needling on spasticity and muscle tone in stroke patients: A systematic review and meta-analysis. Journal of Stroke and Cerebrovascular Diseases. 32(5).

128. Bennett, M.I., Raftery, J. (2019). Central pain mechanisms: understanding the role of sensitization in the management of chronic pain. British Journal of Pain. 13(1): 19-25.

129. Shah, J.P., Thaker, H. (2023). "Nonmyofascial Trigger Points: A Comprehensive Review." Journal of Pain Research. 16: 107-119.

130. Klein, M.J., et al. (2021). "Non-myo-fascial Trigger Points: An Underrecognized Cause of Pain." Journal of Bodywork and Movement Therapies. 25(4): 767-773.

131. Alvarez, D. J., Rockwell, P. G. (2022). "Understanding Non-Myo-Fascial Pain: A Review of Trigger Points and Related Conditions." Pain Medicine. 23(8): 1433-1442.

132. Meyer, M.F., et al. (2022). "Exploring the Mechanisms Behind Dry Needling in Non-myofascial Pain: An Evidence-Based Approach." Clinical Rehabilitation. 36(6): 760-771.

133. Tashjian, R.Z., et al. (2021). "Clinical Approaches to Nonmyofascial Trigger Points." Pain Physician. 24(2): 97-106.

134. Tough, E.A., White, A.R. (2022). "The Role of Dry Needling in Treating Non-Myo-fascial Pain." Current Pain and Headache Reports. 26(6): 455-462.

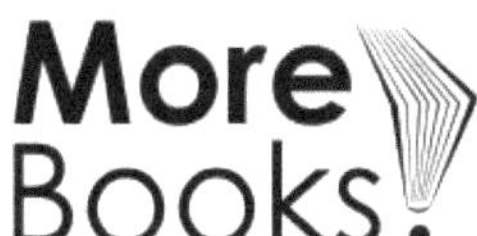

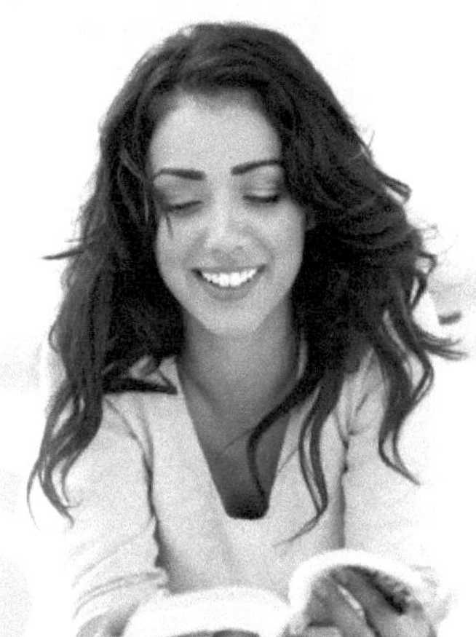

I want morebooks!

Buy your books fast and straightforward online - at one of world's fastest growing online book stores! Environmentally sound due to Print-on-Demand technologies.

Buy your books online at

www.morebooks.shop

Kaufen Sie Ihre Bücher schnell und unkompliziert online – auf einer der am schnellsten wachsenden Buchhandelsplattformen weltweit! Dank Print-On-Demand umwelt- und ressourcenschonend produzi ert.

Bücher schneller online kaufen

www.morebooks.shop

info@omniscriptum.com
www.omniscriptum.com

OMNIScriptum

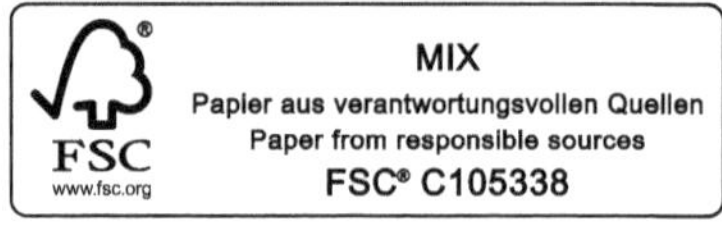

Printed by Books on Demand GmbH, Norderstedt / Germany